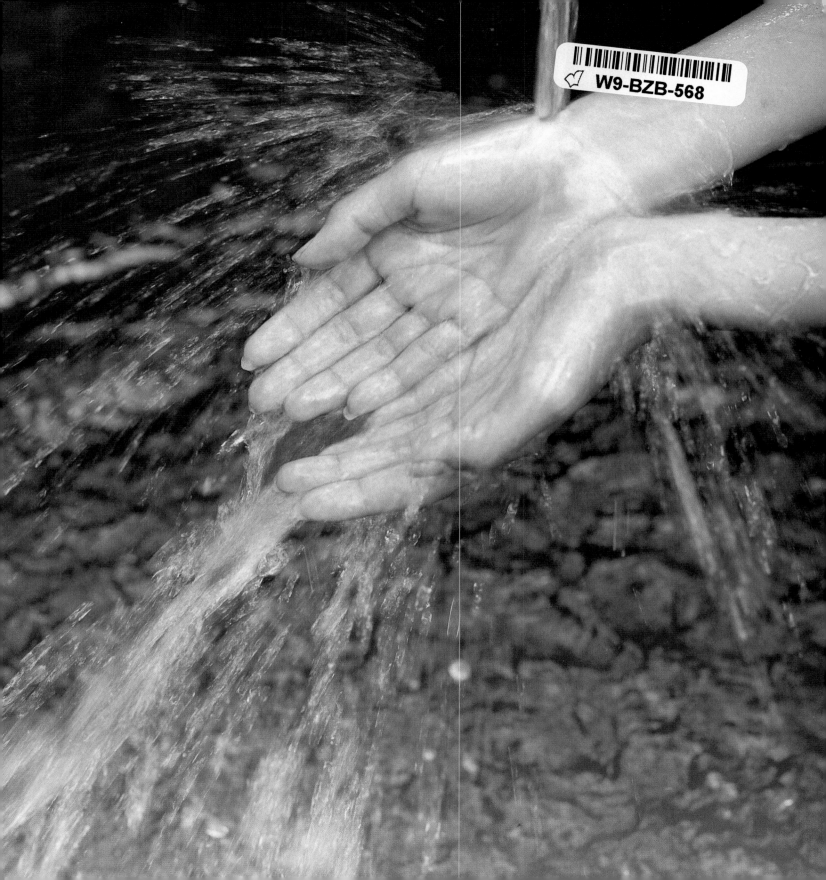

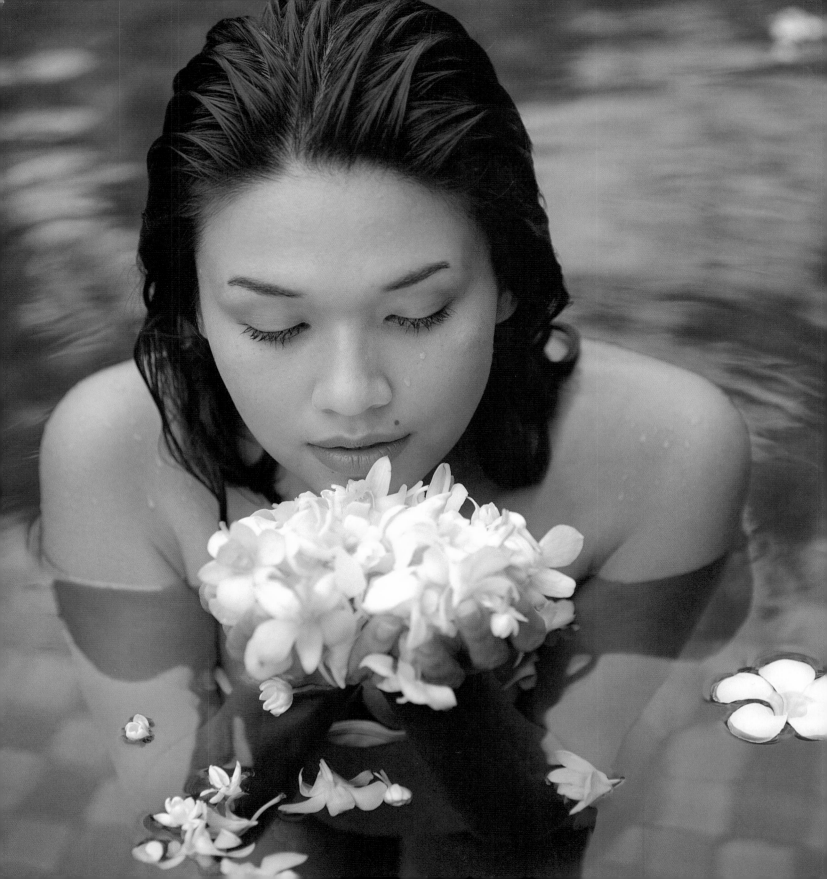

Asian Secrets of
Health, Beauty, and Relaxation

By Sophie Benge
Photos by Luca Invernizzi Tettoni

PERIPLUS

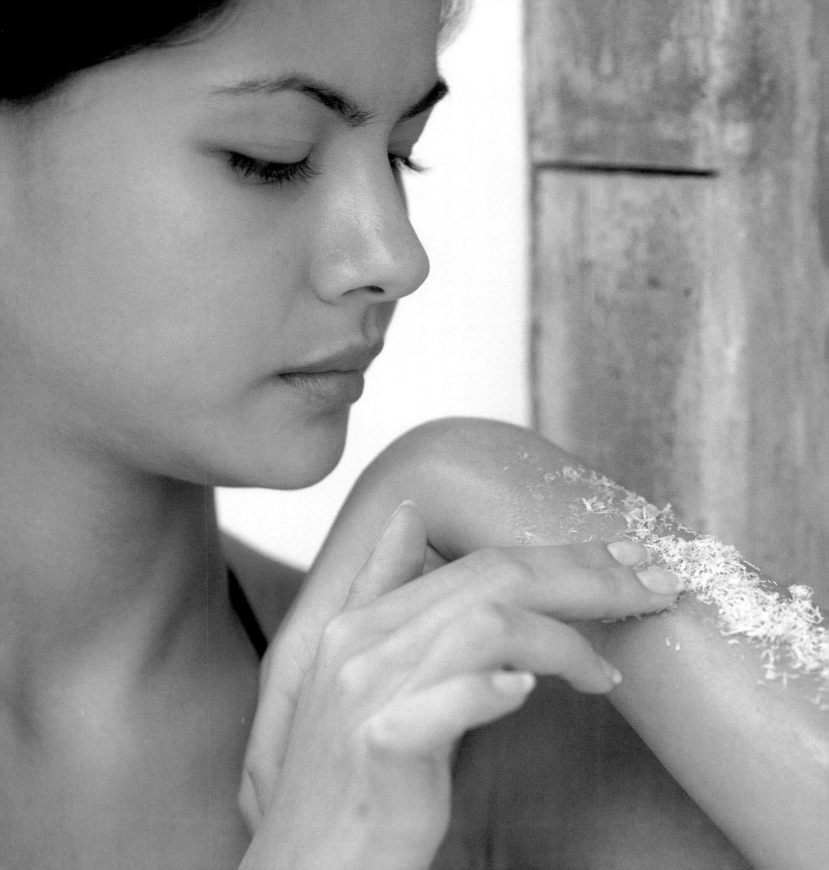

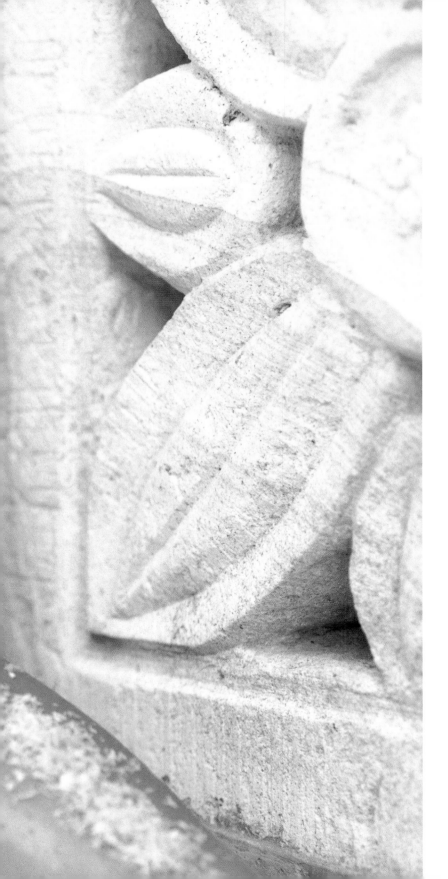

Asian Secrets of Health, Beauty, and Relaxation

Published by Periplus Editions (HK) Ltd
Copyright © 2000 Periplus Editions (HK) Ltd

Publisher: Eric Oey
Associate Publisher: Christina Ong
Editor: Kim Inglis
Designer: Loretta Reilly

The recipes and techniques outlined in *Asian Secrets of Health, Beauty, and Relaxation* are intended for cosmetic and relaxation use only and are not meant to replace diagnosis and treatment by a medical practitioner. Before using any of these recipes, author and publisher recommend consulting a physician. All the recipes have been tested and are considered safe, but since some people have more sensitive skin than others and since the user's actual recipe preparation is beyond the control of the author or publisher, author and publisher accept no liability with regard to the use of recipes or techniques contained in this book.

ISBN 962–593–854-0

Distributed by:
Tuttle Publishing (USA)
364 Innovation Drive
North Clarendon
VT 05759–9436
Toll-free order number 1–800–526–2778
Toll-free fax number 1–800–329–8885

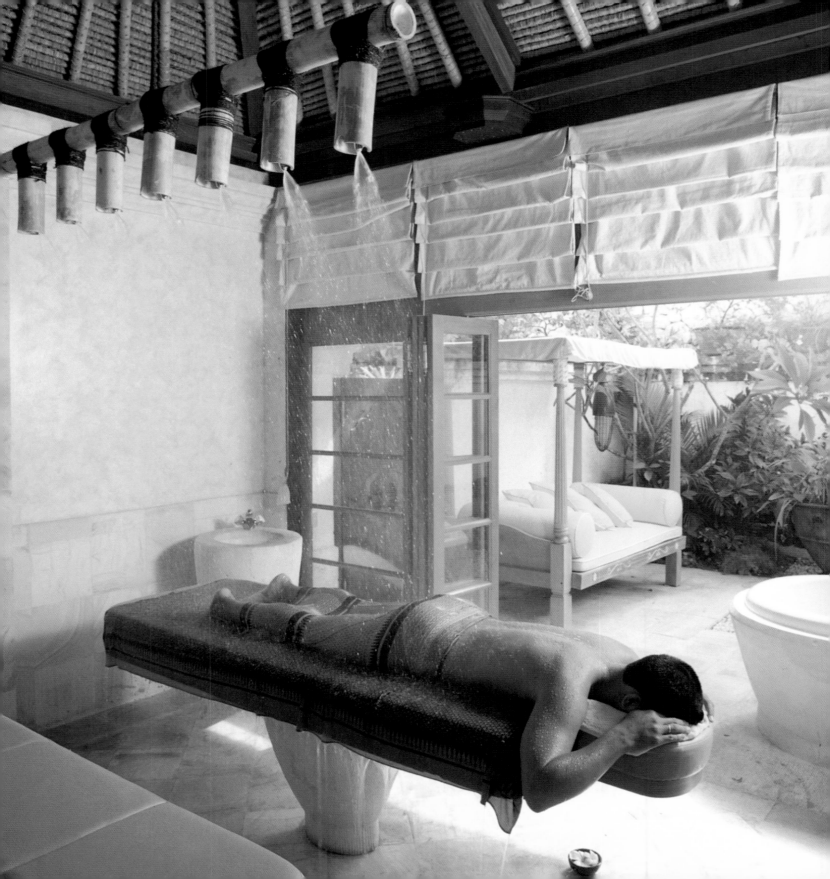

contents

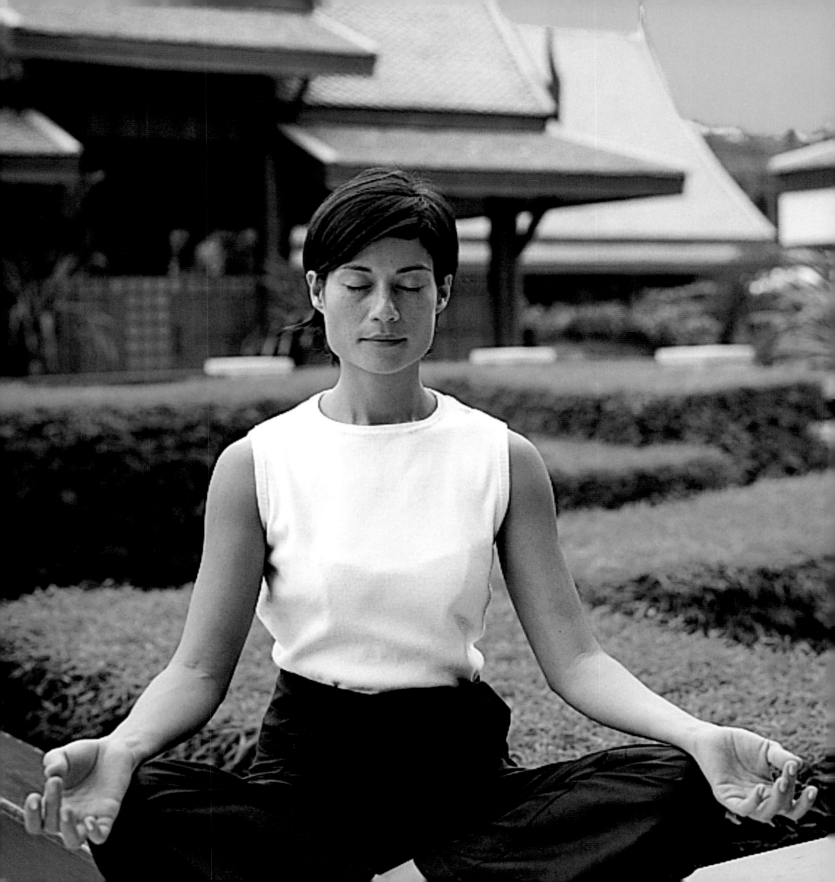

the spa at home

The widespread symbol of Asian philosophy is the circle of yin and yang, where one half flows effortlessly into the other in a synergistic and interlocking whole. Pried apart, these halves are like the quotation marks that open and close a statement; together they are the statement itself.

Just like this ancient symbol, every human being is an interlocking whole whereby spiritual, mental and physical energies flow together to create holistic well-being. Here in America we are just getting comfortable with the concept of holistic thinking, but in Asia it has been at the core of health and beauty customs and practice since the beginning of time. In Java, the birthplace of many Asian health and beauty secrets, this mind-body connection is crystalized by the ancient expression *rupasampat wahya bhiantara*: "the balance between that which is visible and that which lies within".

Mind-body guru Deepak Chopra puts it another way in his best-selling book 'Quantum Healing'. He writes: "The mind and the body are like parallel universes. Anything that happens in the mental universe must leave tracks in the physical one." Indeed, current studies in Western mind-body science have shown that when we are relaxed and happy, the biochemical rhythms in our bodies are significantly different from those present when we are angry, tense or sad.

Physically, we glow when we are feeling well. And when we glow we are beautiful. According to Dr Martha Tilaar, founder and president of one of the Republic of Indonesia's foremost natural cosmetic companies, all the skin and hair products that help cultivate outer beauty are balanced by those for inner beauty such as herbal tonics, exercise, whole food, fasting and selfless gestures toward others. Dr Tilaar reminds us: "This is not religious practice. A sense of gratitude and taking care of others empowers us inside. These actions are part of the beauty ritual." What's more, much Asian ideology says that a desire to be beautiful is valid.

In truth, while *rupasampat wahya bhiantara* may be a foreign phrase, it is certainly not a foreign concept. We know it by expressions such as "beauty comes from within". Too often, though, we're too busy to go beyond the surface, so we gel our hair and reach for some lipstick, dusting on a little outer glow as we dash out the door. When we do try for something deeper, we rush in late to a yogarobics class, feeling too manic to relax properly.

(Page 4–5) The *Spa at Bali Hyatt* mixes its own Asian-based scrubs that are easy to recreate at home – try this dried avocado and coconut exfoliating body scrub.

(Previous page) The *Spa at Jimbaran*, Four Seasons Resort Bali at Jimbaran Bay, is the only tropical spa where you can take a shower lying down. Try replicating somethng similar at home; it feels like gentle rainfall and sends you into a relaxed state.

< A few minutes practising yoga each morning ensures a kickstart to the day.

The spa you create is a sanctuary of the senses, a buffer between timelessness and the stressful urgencies of everyday life.

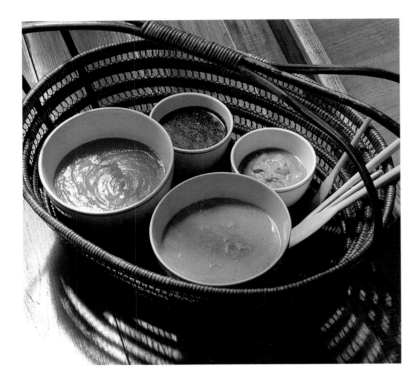

∧ Recipes that smell good enough to eat! Used in Thai massage, these contain sesame oil and seeds, milk, honey and various herbs.

Creating the Asian spa experience at home

The essence of an Asian spa is tranquility, therapy and spirituality packaged in a tropical setting. To lay back amid lush vegetation, perhaps cooled by an ocean breeze, is to let life's stress evaporate slowly from every pore. So you're not in a hut by the ocean? Be inventive, and imagine you are in Bali or Thailand. Substitute the background ebb and flow of the ocean with a CD which plays wave after wave of quiet and splash. You don't even have to get wet to feel refreshed!

Should you choose to take a dip, immerse yourself in the bath. The sensation of floating weightless is primal and powerful. Water, after all, was our first home. To recreate that feeling of warmth, safety and isolation, fill the tub at just about body temperature, and take a relaxing bath. You can maximize its sedative effect with calming oils such as ylang-ylang or sandalwood, and a scented candle at one side. A hot-water soak quickens pulse and induces perspiration, allowing the kidneys to work more efficiently without working harder. Ginger or nutmeg oils enhance relaxation and purification. A hot soak is powerfully soporific, so after 15 minutes or so, you may want to inhale an energizing whiff of peppermint oil to help you climb out of the tub.

So, here's the first secret: Take time for yourself. It sounds simple, but it's easier said than done. One way to do it is to indulge in a spa experience: on vacation or at a day spa, and always with a massage in which you entrust yourself to the gentle hands of another, is one option. Another idea is to recreate the spa experience back at home, where you will find ingredients from your garden to your cupboards, your backyard to your bathroom, which will make a sensual, perhaps spiritual, retreat.

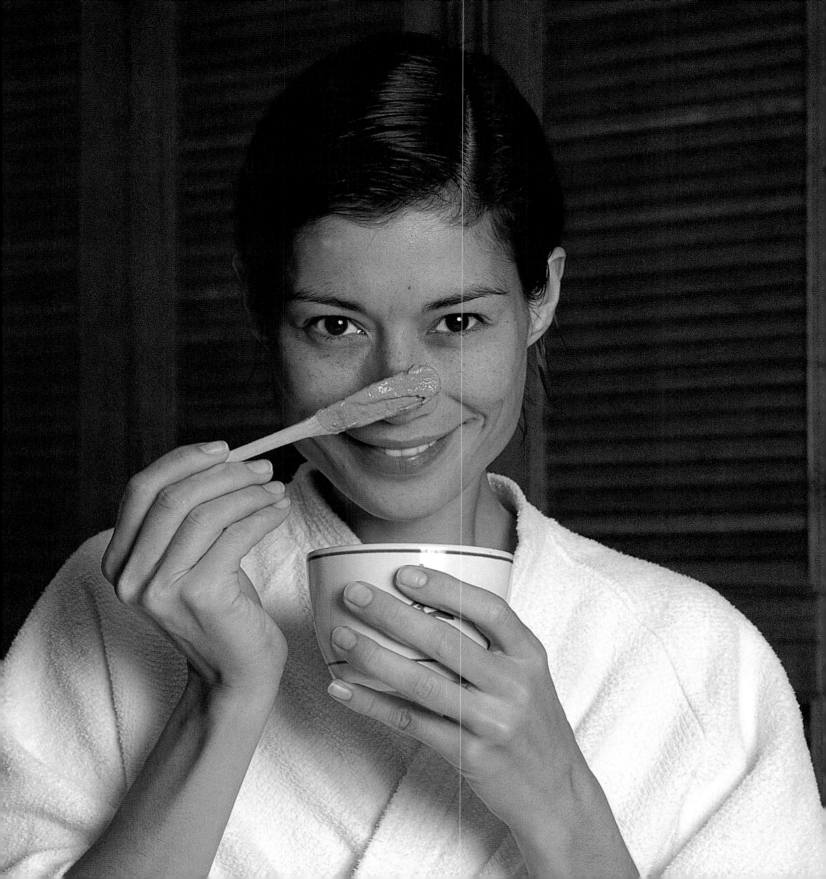

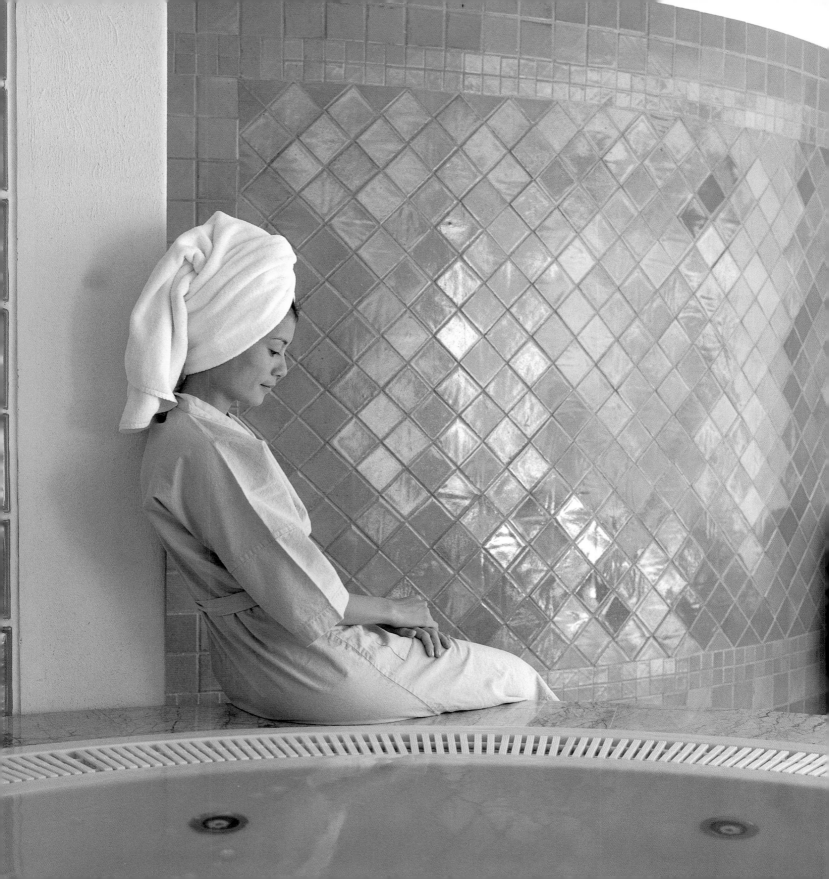

"To make the right choices in life, you need to get in touch with your soul. To do this, you need to experience solitude." *Deepak Chopra*

Alternatively when you take a shower the rainforest you produce in your own bathroom will ease your mind as well as your muscles. The sound of falling water can do that. Music will heighten your sensation. For an Asian mood try the xylophonic rhythms of the Indonesian *gamelan*, the meditative notes of the Japanese *shakuhachi* flute, trance-inducing *qawwali* chants, and the near hypnosis of sitar-based Indian *ragas*. Their harmonics will soothe your rough edges, flushing out the dissonance of tension and filling you with a deep sense of calm. (And, of course, for those deeply rooted in Western tradition, there's always Mozart or some Chopin preludes.)

One of the delights of a tropical spa is the use of outside space. At home, this might be an early-morning dip in the swimming pool before a facial, or an outdoor shower under the stars to wash off a yoghurt rub. Perhaps it's simply a secluded spot under a shady tree in the middle of a Sunday afternoon. So you trade the *bale bengon* – the Javanese daybed – for a webbed chaise longue. Whether inside or outside, the point is you're giving yourself 20 blissful minutes with, perhaps, honey and cucumber on your face, or your hair wrapped in a towel for an aromatherapy scalp treatment – and no one to concentrate on but yourself.

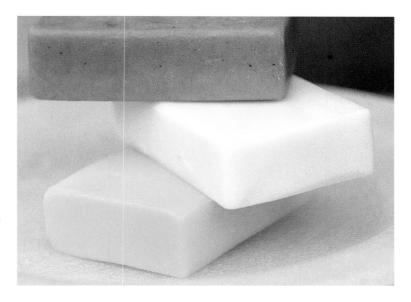

Needless to say the Indonesians have a phrase to describe an experience like this: *leha leha* is a Javanese expression that stands for peace, relaxation, daydreaming, a mind emptied of tension and stress.

A spiritual retreat

The temple of well-being you create in a personal retreat is not only the physical space that encloses your body, but your body itself. Your personal temple takes shape from the inside out. You might, for example, spend a few moments just breathing. Exhale the tensions that have built within you, allowing a

∧ Soaps made in such enticing combinations as Patchouli and Mandarin, Coffee and Pumice, or Clove and Nutmeg are the hallmark of natural bathing.

< Indulge yourself with a relaxing bath before trying a tropical treatment at home.

True tranquility comes from a serene inner core, but burning pachouli, vetiver or clove oils will create an atmosphere thick with calm.

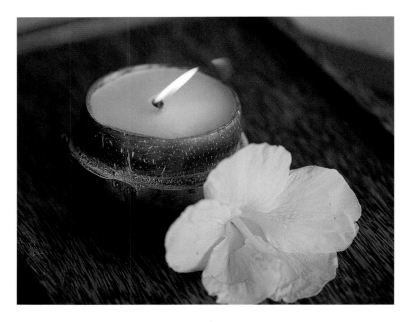

∧ A scented candle and the allure of a tropical bloom can open up the atmosphere to all kinds of possibilities.

> Mindful exercise is integral to the Asian spa philosophy.

cooler, calmer air to enter your lungs. The flame of a candle may help to focus your thoughts – or allow those thoughts to drift away – while a centering fragrance such as sandalwood may create just enough of a veil to separate you, if only for a brief period, from the rest of the world outside.

True tranquility comes from a serene inner core, of course, but burning pachouli, vetiver or clove oils in your bedroom will create an atmosphere thick with calm. The scents themselves may affect you physically. That's the theory behind aromatherapy; it suggests that

the limbic system – the most primal area of the brain responds to scent in a reflexive way. With a whiff of an invigorating scent such as ginger or peppermint, the brain releases endorphins to energize the body. With a calming scent such as vetiver or sandalwood, it releases serotonin, which tells the nervous system to slow down. It is no coincidence that sweet-smelling incense and flowers are abundant in places of worship, where you come to sit quietly and look inward.

But let's return to your own personal temple. "To make the right choices in life, you have to get in touch with your soul. To do this you need to experience solitude," says Deepak Chopra. While you're in the solitary place you have created, why not try chanting? A chant is a form of vocal meditation, a focused combination of sound and breath that resonates in your chest and expands outward through your body, creating a vibrational ripple that extends into the universe.

The simplest and most powerful chant is "Om", the metaphorical sound of the universe. Take a deep breath. On your exhalation, let sound and breath come together. You might say the word in three seamless syllables: *ahhh* from deep within in your chest, *ooooo* as it rises into your throat, and *mmmmm* as the

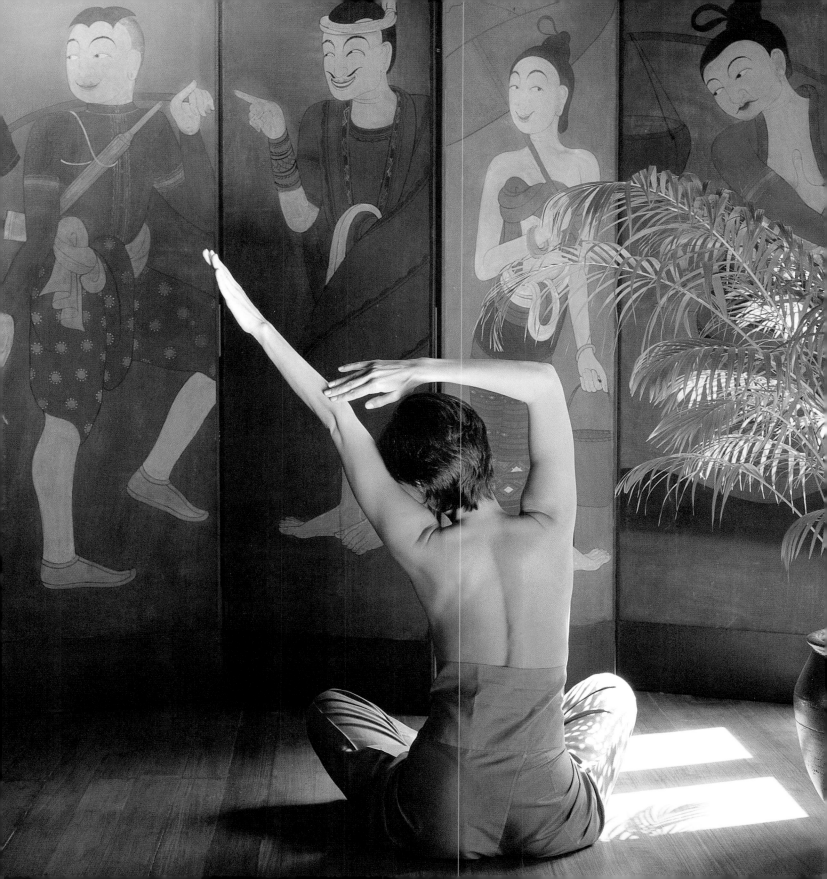

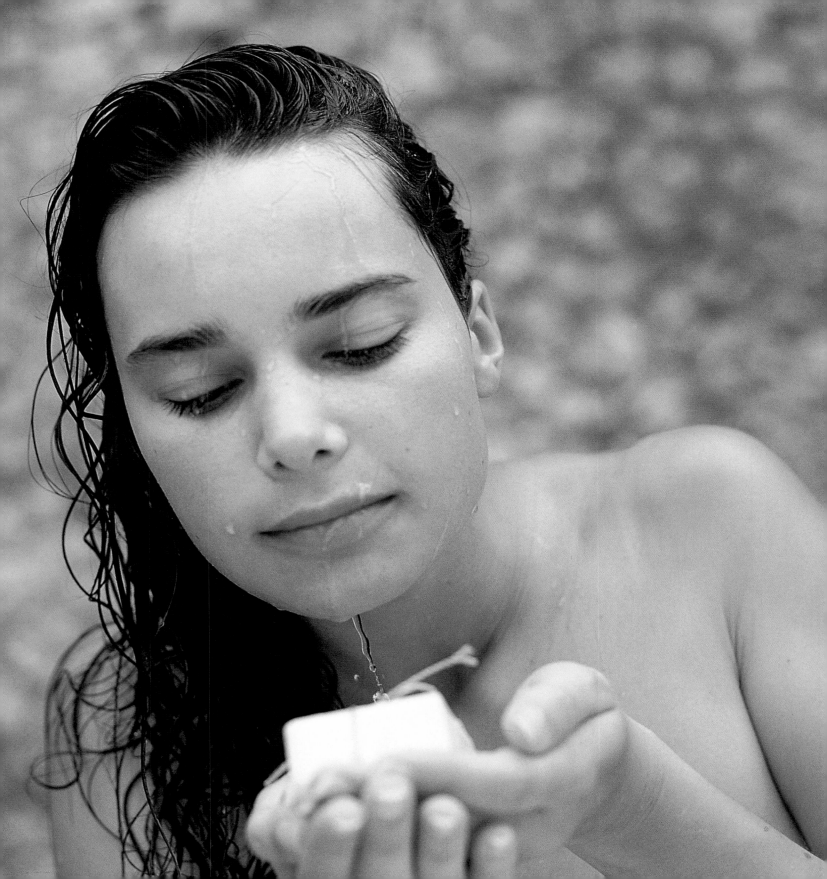

Remember *rupasampat wahya bhiantara:* the balance betrween that which is visible and that which lies within. Complement the inner glow of meditation with the outer glow of exfoliation.

sound exits your mouth and your lips come together. Hold the chant for as long as breath and sound can comfortably travel together. (You'll find that the more you chant, the deeper and longer you are able to do so.)

Those who chant regularly will tell you that sound stimulates the *chakras*, the energy vortexes that exist in the body. The higher *chakras* – those in the chest, throat, forehead and crown – are particularly affected by the vibration of sound and breath. Another secret, then, is that new experiences offer different paths to relaxation.

Yoga is another such path. The benefits of its gentle twists and stretches are effective before, during or after your spa session. If you practice the classic *Salutation to the Sun*, a series of standing and bending *asanas*, or poses, you'll loosen your body in preparation for a soak or scrub. If you're feeling lethargic from a heat treatment, a bit of stretching will energize you. Conversely, if you find you're not as relaxed as you'd like to be during your spa session, mindful movement will help release tension. With the pliable muscles of a relaxed body you'll find it easier to extend into stretches that are normally difficult. If you're new to yoga, your spa-loose limbs will allow you to experiment with the poses more freely.

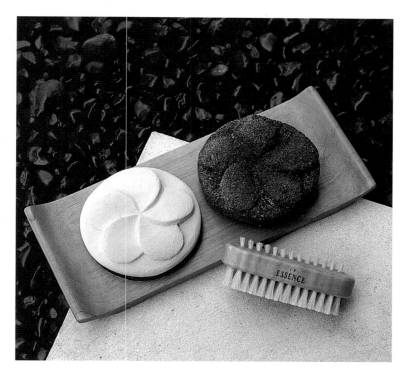

You will likely come away from even a few moments of chanting or stretching with a fuller heart, a clearer head, and a body pleasantly free of tension. So cleansed, you may feel that a Honey-Cucumber Mask for your face or a Kemiri Nut Scrub for your feet is beside the point. But remember *rupasampat wahya bhiantara.* Why not complement the inner glow of meditation with the outer glow of exfoliation? It is easy enough to organize in your own home.

∧ Pumice, scrubs and even brushing the skin are good for exfoliation.

< Smell is our most neglected sense; the feelings evoked by the scent of a soap or candle can be very powerful.

"Thai massage is a healing experience for the giver as well as the receiver and intrinsic life energy will flow between the two." *Khun Sutthichai Teimeesak, chief massage therapist at the Oriental Spa, Bangkok*

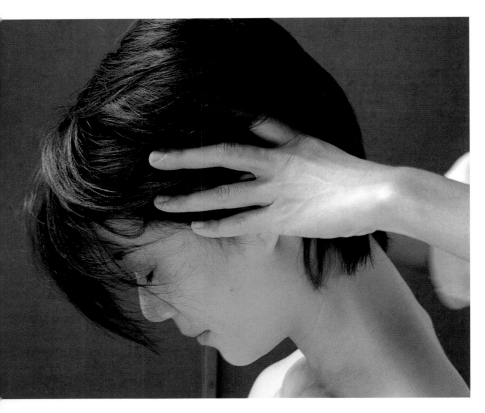

^ The head is a key zone in Thai massage. Pressure along the scalp lines can increase blood flow to the head as many of the body's nerves congregate here.

Spa therapists make their clients feel special through attention and touch. This is exactly what we do for our partners, and what they in turn do for us. Combining intimacy with therapy is a wonderful way to escape together. Not only does it give you tranquil time away from the bedroom, it expands the range of spa options, because now you have someone to rub your temples, massage your feet or, for example, administer an Aloe and Lavender Wrap to every square inch of your body.

Traditional massage is one of the most important aspects of the Asian spa regime, because it embodies the essence of yin and yang. "Massage is a healing experience for the giver as well as the receiver, and life energy will flow between the two," says Khun Sutthichai Teimeesak, chief massage therapist at Bangkok's *Oriental Spa*. What's more, the time away from pressing concerns will strengthen the bonds between you both as it loosens your individual or shared tensions.

Sharing your spa experience

We began by suggesting you try a solitary spa experience, because with a schedule full of appointments and family obligations, sometimes all you want is a little bit of peace and quiet by yourself. But sharing your spa time — with a partner or a friend or even a small group — can be just as fun.

The communal bath has long been a feature of civilization, from the Roman *therma* to the Finnish *sauna*, the Turkish *hamam* to the Japanese hot tub. With that in mind, why not invite your closest girlfriends over for an afternoon of aqueous bonding and indulgent spa treatments? There may be more serene ways

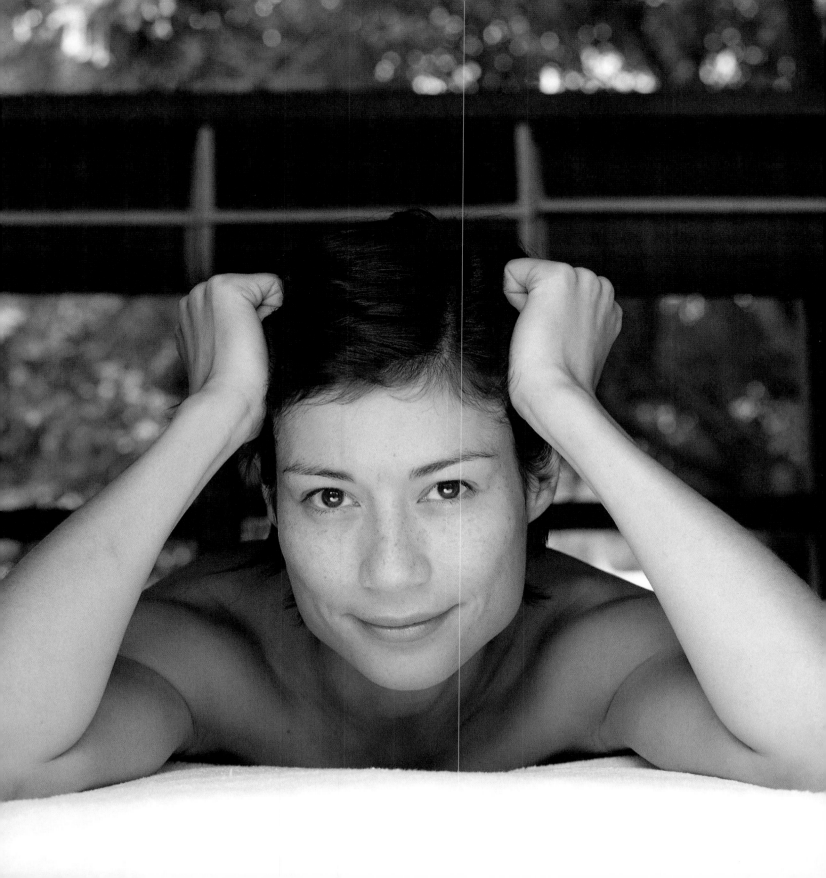

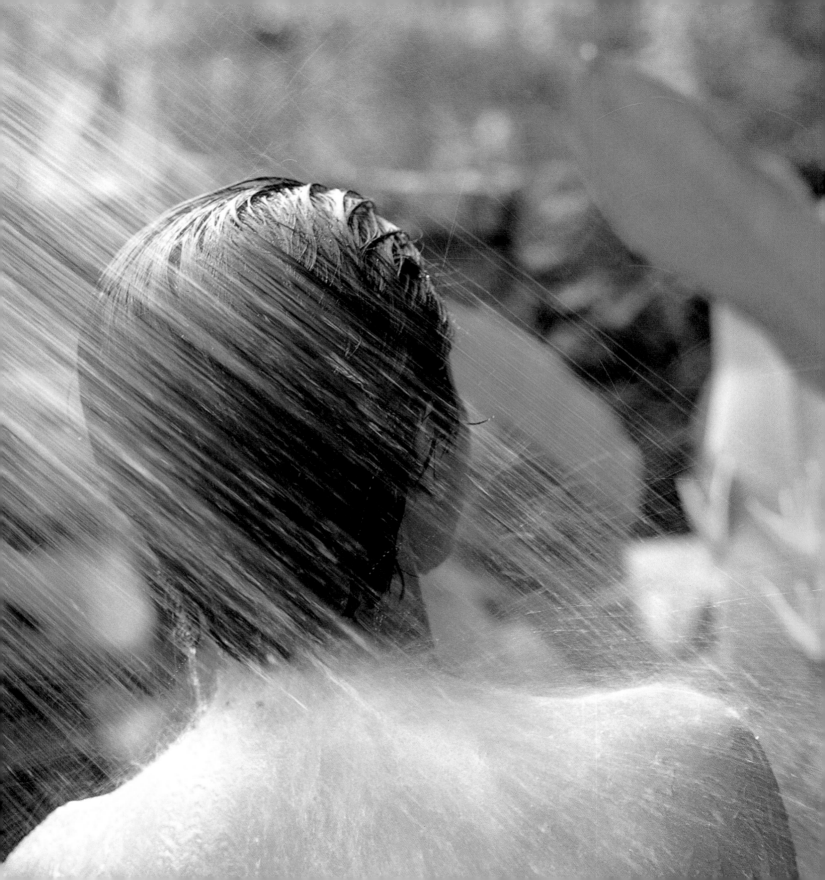

Why not invite your closest girlfriends over for an afternoon of aqueous bonding and indulgent spa treatments? There may be more serene ways to experience mind-body healing, but they won't be as much fun.

to experience mind-body healing, but they won't be as enjoyable. Besides, who else would be willing to spend three hours with you perched on the side of the tub wrapped in a towel? And who else would you permit to see you in a rice-powder mask? If you have access to a backyard pool or an outdoor shower, all the better.

You'll heighten the camaraderie with the scent of jasmine. Throughout Asia it is the fragrance of friendship and femaleness. You might also take a cue from one of Bali's top spas and break halfway through the afternoon with cool fruit drinks or herbal teas and a fruit plate prepared beforehand.

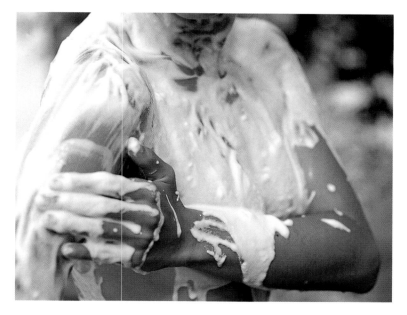

Food for the body, inside and out

What better way is there to appreciate the harmony of health, beauty and the natural world than by transforming fresh foodstuffs into natural treatments? Many of the spa ingredients in this book are easily found in your local supermarket, if they are not already in your cupboard: turmeric and ginger, honey and sesame seeds, for instance. Also, foods no longer need to be in season to be available. Tropical fruits such as avocado, papaya, coconut and lime are easily found year-round. Hard-to-find items are often available from

specialist Asian grocery stores. Even in mid-size cities, you'll find such exotic items as lemon grass and galangal, a rhizome in the ginger family. Then there are the ingredients you can grow yourself, in pots on the kitchen counter or in a small plot in the backyard: aloe and mint, for example. Your intuition will guide you as to what's right for you. It may be honey or mud, sea salt or clay.

Another pleasure of a home spa is the smell, taste and feel of your treatments – familiar foods with new and slightly exotic sensations. A trickle of cucumber pulp between the toes

∧ The final stage of a Javanese Lulur involves an all-over body splash with natural yoghurt – go on, enjoy!

< Outdoor showers are an integral part of the tropical spa experience; try to recreate that sensation at home.

The temple of well-being you create in a personal spa retreat is not only the physical space that encloses your body, but your body itself.

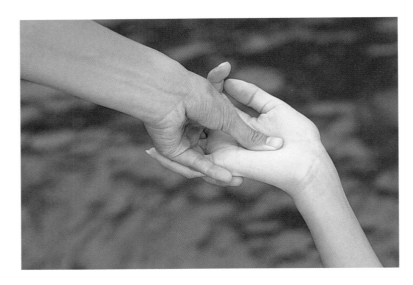

∧ Hand movements in traditional Balinese massage.

> Splash out and enjoy the benefits of fresh water.

beats rubbing cream into your heels. The heat of cloves and ginger smeared over your shoulder or the pungent smell of coffee bean wafting up from your cleavage elicits a sensuous shiver of delight. Moreover, the effect of some of these traditional whole food treatments is grounded in science. For example, the *lulur* or body treatment with its all-over yoghurt body splash or the Payaya Body Polish puréed from whole fruit, contain mild acids that are akin to the alpha hydroxy acids (AHAs) we've seen touted on the pages of women's magazines at stratospheric prices. Milk and fruit acids loosen the bonds between dead skin and the live layer beneath it. Exfoliate with a loofah or terry towel and you'll reveal glowing skin with

a smoother texture and more uniform color. The benefit of a whole-food treatment is that it is gentle and gradual. You will be unlikely to experience any irritation on contact with the skin as you may with the concentrated commercial product (just be sure to rinse off your treatment entirely before going in the sun). And, of course, it *feels* as luscious as it looks.

The elements of the Asian spa

Whether you go halfway around the world to relax or create the experiences at home, you'll draw on the same basic elements – water, air, fire and earth.

Water – fresh or saline – hot, warm or cool... water is restorative and purgative. Water has been the essence of a traditional spa since ancient times. Immersion is the sum and substance of ritual purification in most religions, for water is the most powerful yet soothing element on earth. According to Hindu legend, *tirtha* or holy water is carried from the sea by a beautiful goddess and drunk to obtain immortality. Lakshmi, the Hindu goddess of good fortune rose from the foam, and as she did, so the rivers changed course to flow toward her. The Chinese Kuan-Yin, known as Kannon in Japan, is goddess of water and the moon; she is often depicted sitting on a lotus

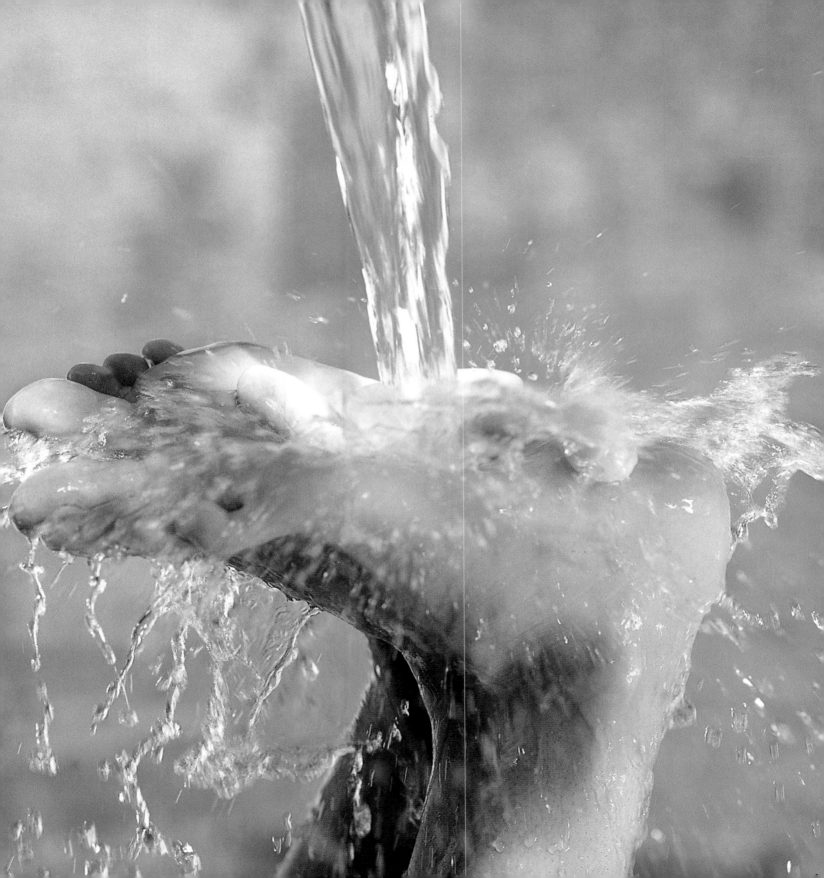

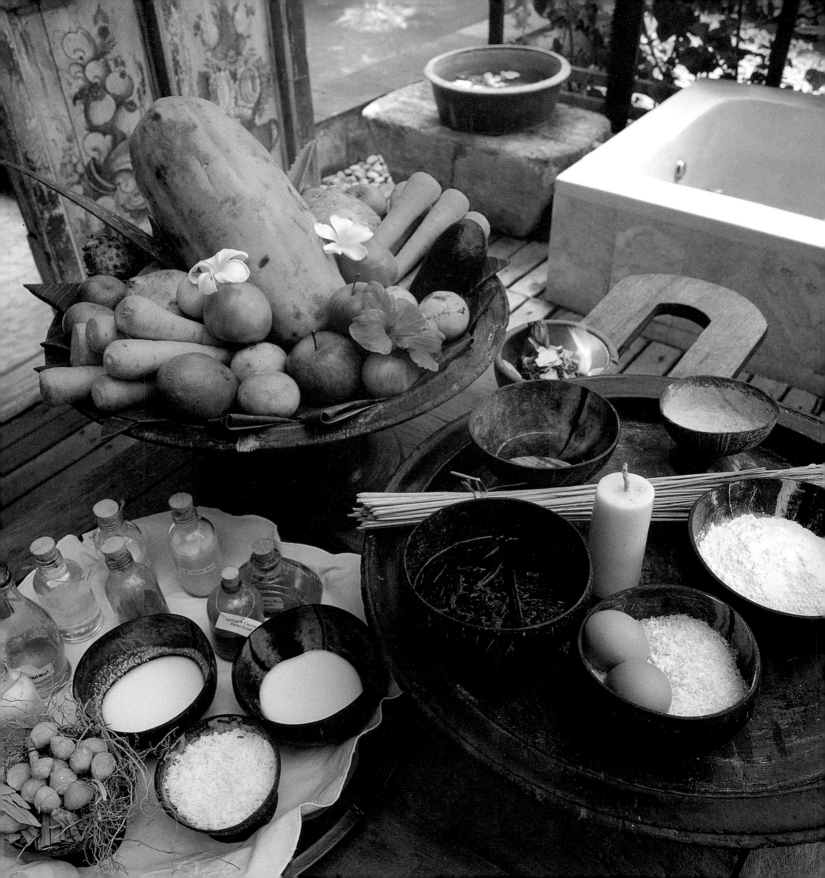

What better way is there to appreciate the harmony of health, beauty and the natural world than by transforming fresh foodstuffs into natural treatments?

blossom, a pure, water-rooted flower that symbolizes enlightenment. Lakshmi and Kuan-Yin are undoubtedly related to the Yoruba goddess Yemaya, ruler of the rivers and seas, and Aphrodite or Venus, the Greco-Roman deity who was borne of the ocean. In Botticelli's famous painting, *The Birth of Venus,* she rises up fully formed on a shell. After a long spa soak, you may rise from the tub feeling something like that yourself.

Scenting the air is the easiest way to create a spa mood at home, for a fragranced atmosphere – whether from burning oil or incense – enhances your sense of well-being at the first moment you inhale. But taking a few moments to breathe consciously will allow you to really center and thus benefit more deeply from your spa experience. Conscious breathing is different from normal breathing. The latter comes instinctively. To breathe consciously you become aware of your rhythm: lungs filling with air, ribcage expanding, body filling with the energy of that inhalation; then the reverse, letting go but without losing that energy.

In Oriental philosophy, breath is synonymous with inspiration from the gods, so it is no wonder that mind-body activities such as yoga and meditation focus on conscious breathing. Air is breath, and breath is life. From yoga to

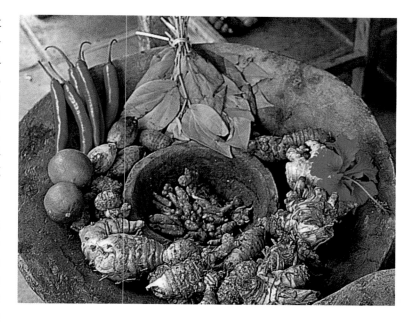

tai-chi to chanting, conscious breathing helps us relax into calmness as still as a lake or, conversely, helps us tap into the rushing rivers of energy. The *chi* of tai chi means "vital breath", as does the *ki* of aikido and the *qi* of qi gong. In yogic philosophy, it is *prana*, the life energy that unites us with one another and with the whole universe.

Fire is another of the primal elements and its benefits have been used in many different cultures for purification purposes. While roaring flames don't figure into the spa experience, the pinpoint of light emitted by a

∧ A selection of roots and rhizomes used in the preparation of traditional treatments at the *Tugu Spa* in Bali.

< You may dip into nature's store cupboard in order to make some of the tantalizing natural treatments offered here.

"If you want skin that is irresistible to the touch, the secret is to touch yourself,"
Pratima Raichur, Ayurvedic physician

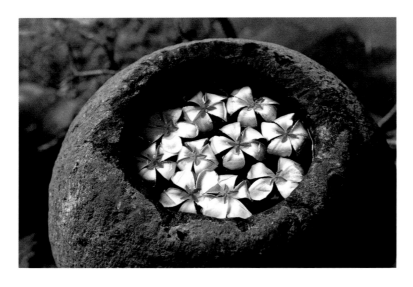

∧ Exotic blooms
are part of the
Asian spa culture:
floral baths, foot
soaks or a simple
flower arrange-
ment floating in
water heighten
the senses.

> A dip before
or after a treat-
ment is an all-
round revitalizer.

Many of the natural reatments that are now commonly used throughout tropical Asian countries trace their origins to the palaces of Central Java. From the 17th century until today, princesses from Solo, Yogyakarta and Surakarta have experimented with natural potions of their own making. Some remedies remain safely hidden behind palace walls. Others, such as the Javanese Lulur, have found their way around the region, and even the world. This famous body scrub of rice, spices and splashes of natural yoghurt is a skin-softening elixir that eclipses the best commercially available body creams. In this book we also include treatments composed from clay, mud and salt.

burning candle provides a most effective means of centering yourself. More dramatically, an array of candles in a darkened room can transform familiar surroundings, an effect heightened by the burning of fragrance. Don't forget the heat sensation from a poultice, such as the Thai Herbal Heat Revival, or even the warm comfort produced by the friction of skin against skin in massage.

Then there are flowers. For all Asian people, flowers are part of everyday life, right down to ablutions. If a rose-petal bath is impossible (and unfortunately urban plumbing may prohibit such a sublime sensation) you have essential flower oils to recreate the fragrance and luxury of a floral bath. Consider the blossom-based treatments of Balinese culture, and then recreate them for yourself using the recipes in this book: a floral foot soak at the start of each treatment, a massage with flower-based essential oils, an aromatherapy scalp treatment, and finally live blossoms woven into the hair.

Radiant skin and shiny hair have been created from Asia's vast botanical heritage. On the Indonesian island of Java alone 6,500 species of plant have been recorded. Malaysia lays claim to 3,600 species of tree, and other tracts of rainforest still wait to be discovered.

Is there anything headier?

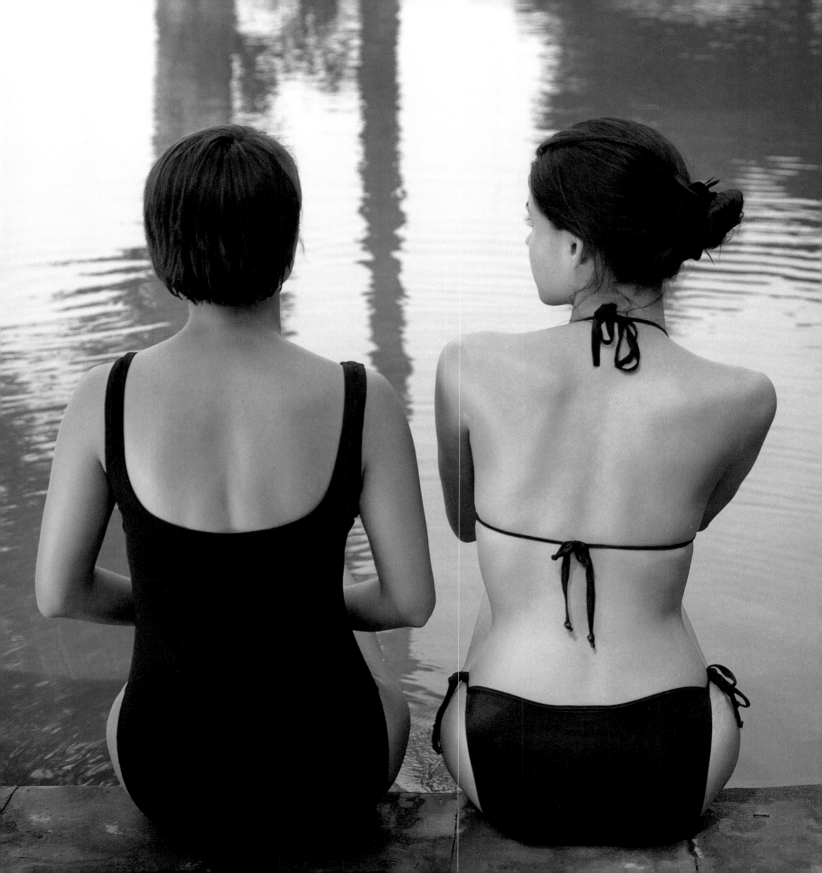

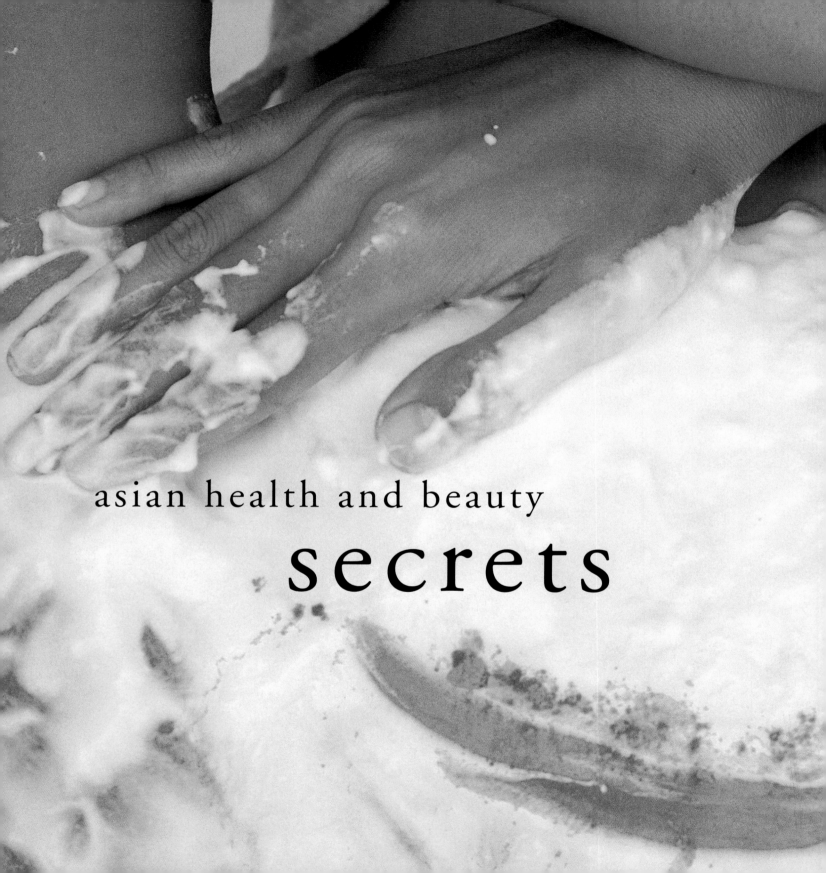

asian health and beauty
secrets

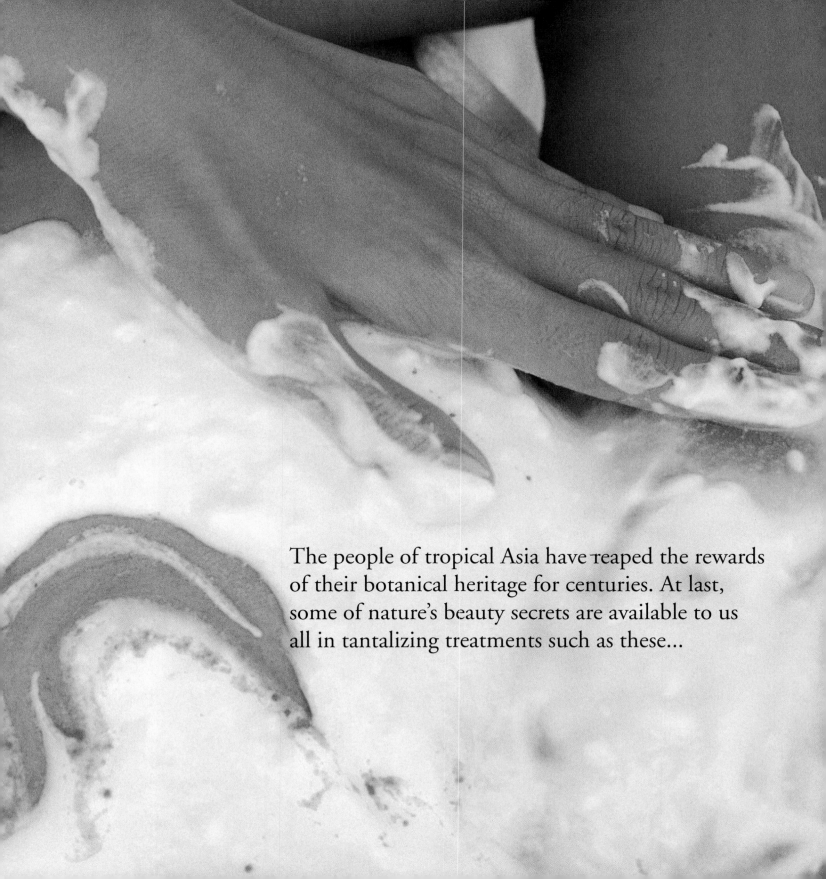

The people of tropical Asia have reaped the rewards of their botanical heritage for centuries. At last, some of nature's beauty secrets are available to us all in tantalizing treatments such as these...

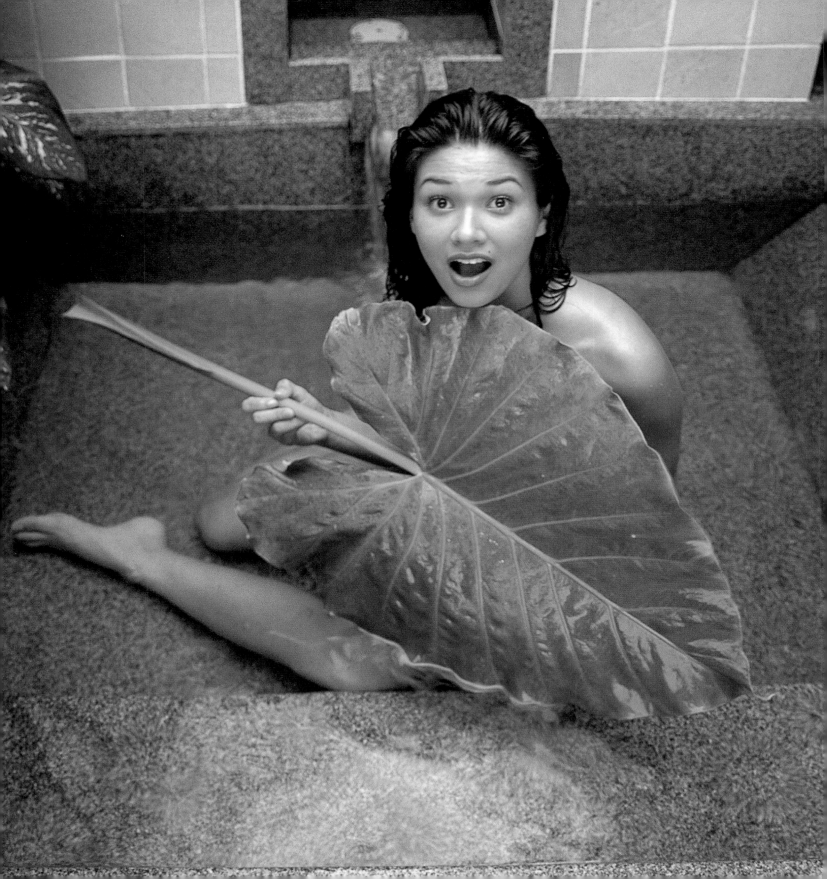

body conscious

Long limbs and vital statistics are minor contributors to the beautiful body. Much more important is the state of mind that sits on top. While there is barely a woman alive who is content with her natural shape, every woman can improve her body by upping the respect that she pays to it. This is achieved by taking time for herself – a vital part of life that most of us ignore.

The Asian approach to achieving and maintaining a healthy and beautiful body is a sensible one. For a start, it has no time for fad diets and punishing stomach crunches! Traditional body treatments from the tropics outstrip those from everywhere else in the world in number and variety and all of them rely on nature's own pharmacopoeia to produce results. Certainly not skin deep, they not only cleanse and soften our skin, but also draw out impurities from within. Their ritual of application (especially at the hands of dedicated therapists in a spa context) relaxes us, empties our minds and soothes our souls in an atmosphere of peace.

All this emphasizes the oriental philosophy that regards beauty as a holistic concept embracing both the inner and outer self. For example, there are everyday words in the Indonesian language that are part of the more specific lexicon of body care which have no real equivalent in English. Indonesian women talk about having a *lulur* or *mangir* or *mandi susu* as readily as westerners talk of taking a shower. This chapter reveals some of the more exotic body treatments, be they scrubs, baths, wraps, heat treatments and polishes, for glowing skin... and improved self-esteem!

Mandi Susu

The tale of Queen Cleopatra and her milk baths is well known, yet do you know anyone who pours a few pints into the tub before climbing in? Trust the Indonesian people with their deep grasp of the good of the natural, to have their own form of milk bath. Known as *Mandi Susu*, it has soaked Javanese princesses for centuries as an elixir of eternal youth. Milk, from a goat, sheep or cow, makes skin radically soft and pure to the touch.

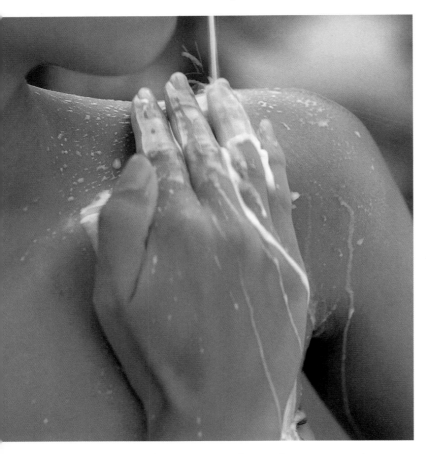

Modern formulations of this popular ritual have eliminated the taste and smell of milk while maintaining its nutrients with softening proteins. The *Mandi Susu* is a sought-after bathing ritual at the *St Gregory Javana Spa* in Singapore where therapists leave you soaking in a cloudy white tub for 20 minutes and advise you not to rinse afterwards. At home, you can pour fresh or powdered milk in with the bath water. Or for superior baby-soft skin, try natural yoghurt or buttermilk, but be ready to hold your nose!

Ocean Bath

This bath focuses on the healing properties of unrefined sea salt harvested on the east coast of Bali. Although not strictly thalassotherapy, this bath relies on the nutrients in the salt to draw out toxins from the body. The benefit of sea salt is based on the premise that sea-water has practically the same chemical make-up as human plasma allowing the body to easily absorb its healing properties.

The Ocean Bath at *The Spa at Jimbaran*, Four Seasons Resort, Bali is altogether a more exotic affair. Not only are the pure sea salts mixed with Bali Sunset Oil containing coconut, vanilla and citrus blends to uplift the senses, this hour-long treatment kicks off with a scalp, neck, shoulder and back massage. As if that were not enough, it takes place in the privacy of your own villa, where the bath tubs have earned an international reputation for their depth, size and comfort.

Floral Bath

For those of us born outside tropical Asia, the floral bath is the nub of the 'tropical spa' experience. We can hardly believe our eyes when a bucket of vivid blooms is tossed into the water purely for our pleasure. It is a sybaritic moment when the velvety petals tickle our bare skin. Flowers – jasmine, gardenia, tropical magnolia, hibiscus, frangipani, bougainvillea, poinciana, rose, globe amaranth, alamanda and ylang-ylang – are chosen both for their fragrance and rich colours.

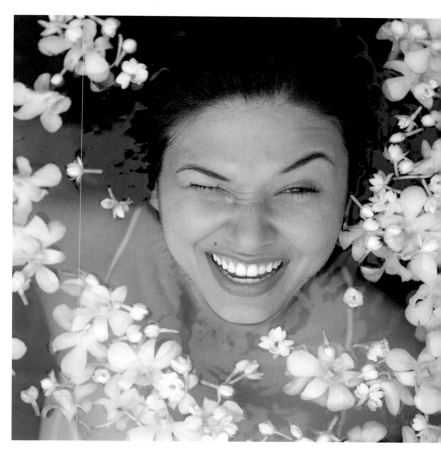

In line with tropical mores, Asians believe flowers are the tangible link to the forces of the spiritual world, representing a symbolic purge of our earthly impurities. In Asian spas, the Floral Bath is not usually offered as a treatment on its own. It is often used as the finale to one of the many tropical body treatments on the menu. It becomes an opportunity to savour the cleansing experience and relax for a further 20 minutes or so.

Aromatherapy Bath

The bath is a perfect place to enjoy the sensual pleasures of aromatherapy oils. Simply drop one or a combination of essential oils into warm water and spuddle. Some of the oils' properties are absorbed into the skin while the rest evaporate into the atmosphere for inhaling, simultaneously soothing muscles and mind.

A Few Recommended Bathtime Blends
Use up to ten drops of these essential oils either together or separately.

For calming	camomile, lavender, rose
For detoxifying	ginger, sage, rosemary
For passion	ylang-ylang, geranium, sandalwood
For brain boosting	grapefruit, lemon, mandarin, peppermint, pine

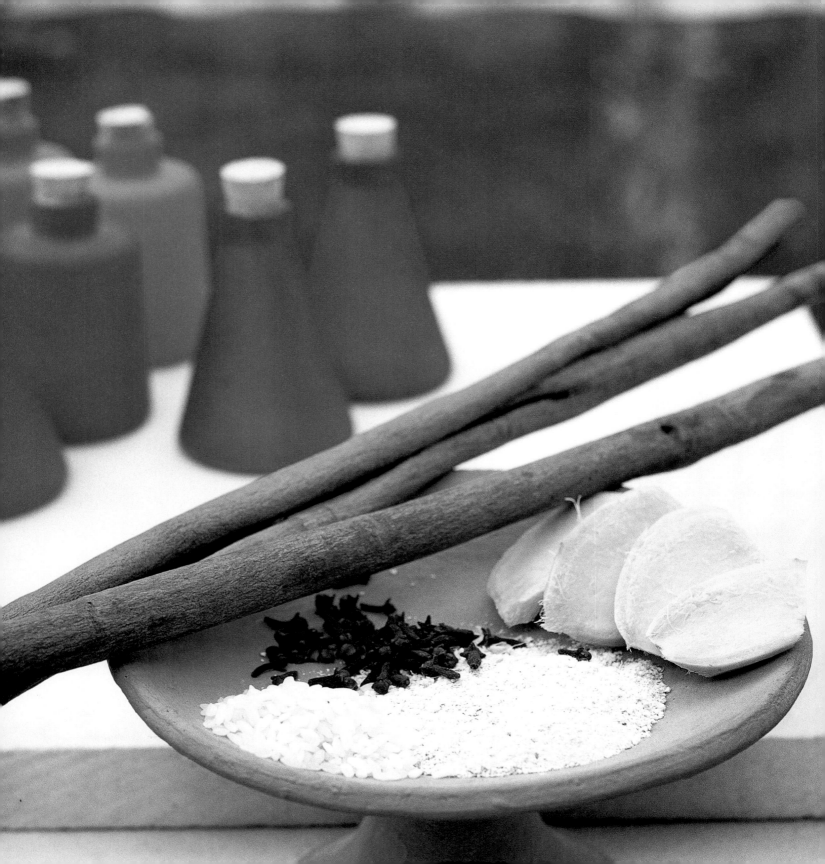

Balinese Boreh

If you reach for the Vicks pot at a hint of a chesty cough, this body scrub is for you. Out of all the oriental treatments the Balinese Boreh offers the most potent sensation – an all-over deep heat experience. The scrub is purely and simply a herb and spice mix: It is a centuries-old village recipe using spices we more readily associate with curry, and is prepared to warm the body at the first sign of windy weather.

As a tropical people, the Balinese live in fear of the cold and the health problems it can bring, so the whole family has a *boreh* both as a curative and preventative treatment. It feels really hot; it's good for fever, headaches, muscle aches, arthritis and chills. It increases the blood circulation and its exfoliating ingredients -- cloves and rice – soften the skin.

The *boreh* is not recommended for pregnant women as the penetrative ingredients direct the heat away from the womb area to the body's extremities.

While most Balinese spas offer the *boreh*, this recipe comes from the *Nusa Dua Spa*.

Ingredients

20 gms (4 tsp)	sandalwood
10 gms (2 tsp)	whole cloves
10 gms (2 tsp)	ginger
5 gms (1 tsp)	cinnamon
10 gms (1 tsp)	coriander seeds
10 gms (1–2 tsp)	rice powder (finely ground rice)
5 gms (1 tsp)	turmeric
10 gms (1 tsp)	nutmeg
10 gms (1 tsp)	lesser galangal water or spice-blended oil
3	large carrots, grated

The first eight ingredients are ground together in a pestle and mortar or bought prepared in powder form or dried in balls.

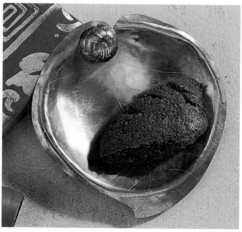

Steps

1   Add a little water or a spice-blended oil to the herb and spice mix to make a thick paste. For those who cannot tolerate a strong heat sensation, mix a greater proportion of ground rice powder to reduce intensity.
2   Cover your body; leave for five to ten minutes; feel the heat!
3   Rub the skin vigorously so that the mixture flakes away.
4   Gently rub the grated carrot into the skin. This replenishes moisture after exfoliating.
5   Shower and moisturize.

Volcanic Clay Body Scrub for Cellulite

Sadly there is no quick fix for beating that orange peel look that decorates the thighs of 95 percent of women. Improved diet, drinking water, dry skin brushing, swimming and yoga all help. And luckily the volcanic island of Bali is home to mineral-rich clays, which seep into the skin to break down those fat cells that are packed in a mattress effect underneath. A good cellulite treatment is the Volcanic Clay Body Scrub at the *Nusa Dua Spa*.

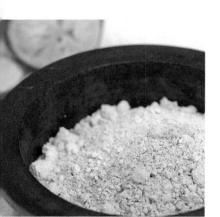

Ingredients

25 gms (2 tbsp)	Balinese clay (or any clay with purifying properties)
30 gms (2 tbsp)	sea salt
	water

Steps

1. Mix ingredients together, adding a little water to make a light paste.
2. Wipe cursorily over entire body. It leaves a thin, white film and feels prickly as it penetrates the skin.
3. Once the paste is dry, rub the skin so that it is sloughed away.
4. Shower and massage. The best essential oils for cellulite are nutmeg and rose. Add a few drops to a carrier oil or your favourite body cream, and apply liberally.

Cucumber Wrap for Sunburnt Skin

Feel the heat seep out of your sunburnt body using cucumber and essential oils. The best Cucumber Cooling Wrap is offered at the *Spa at Bali Hyatt*. Here's their recipe.

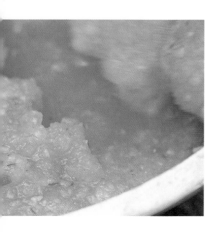

Ingredients

2 kilos (4 lb)	cucumbers, plus skin and pips, whizzed in a blender
2 drops	lavender oil
2 drops	tea tree oil
2 drops	camomile oil

Steps

1. Cover your body with the cucumber mixed with the essential oils.
2. Wrap the body in a gauze or cotton sheet; leave for 30 minutes.
   The cucumber feels cool on tender skin and you can sense the heat being drawn out of your body.
3. Cucumber leaves the skin soft, so moisturizing afterwards is optional.

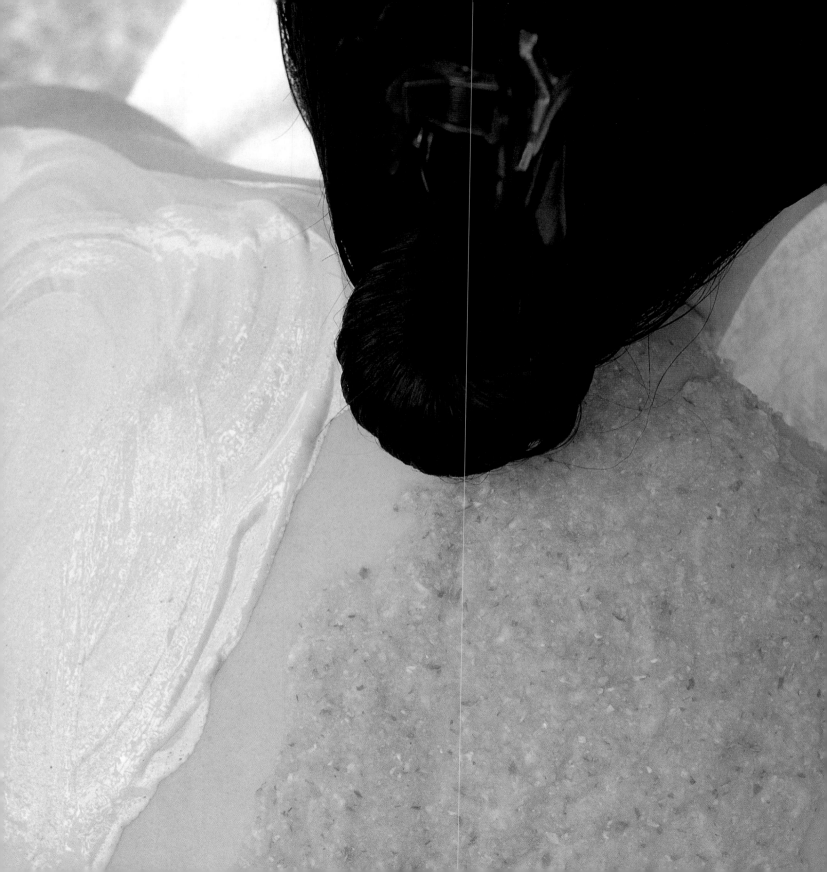

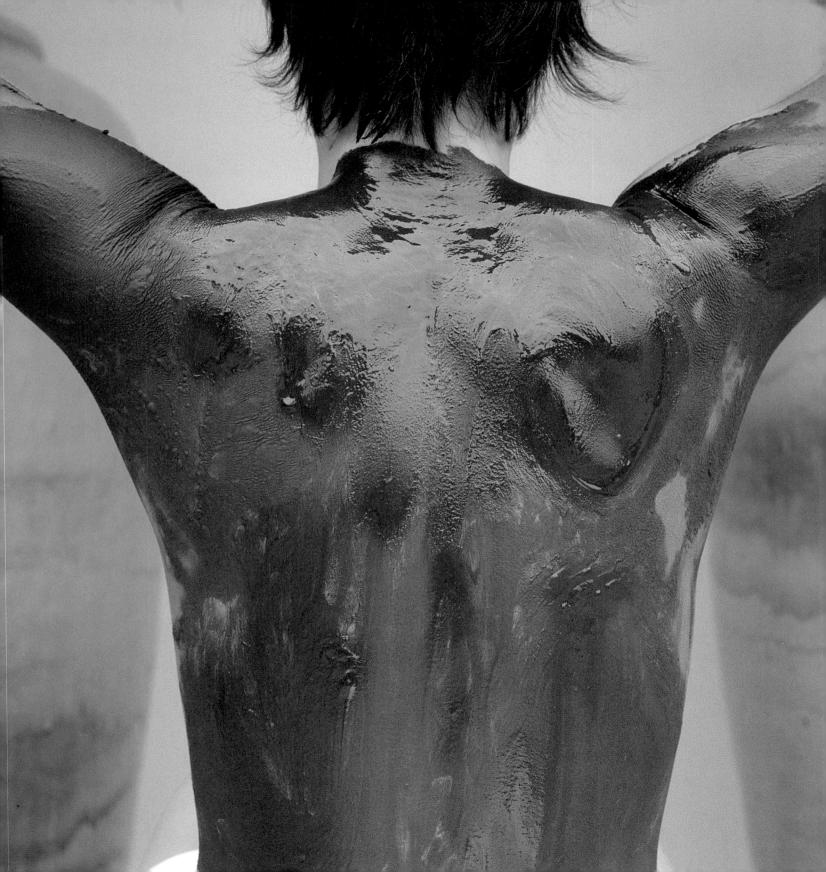

Thai Herbal Wrap

Enjoy this soft and aromatic body wrap only in Thailand where the healing properties of the country's mineral-rich mud remain both a mystery and a secret.

For a particularly seductive herbal wrap, which looks and smells more suitable for the dinner table than the body, visit *The Oriental Spa*, Bangkok. Here the hotel chef mixes a closely guarded recipe of white Thai mud, milk and turmeric, herbs and sesame oil which smells divine and feels soft and silky when applied to the skin.

Your body is wrapped in a plastic sheet, topped with towels while the creamy Thai mud concoction draws out any infection and impurities from the body and heals blemishes on the skin's surface. After perspiring gently for 20 minutes, take a shower, pat dry and feel the smooth, satin texture of your skin. There is no need to moisturize.

Alternatively the magic mud mixture used for the wrap at *Chiva-Som* (opposite) is dark and viscous like treacle. It feels warm and velvety on the skin and likewise is applied over the entire body, which is wrapped in a plastic sheet and covered with towels. This mud comes from the north of the country and is mixed with turmeric, marjoram and natural spring water.

Din So Porng (White Thai Mud)

Before the advent of deodorant sticks and Evian water sprays, the Thai people had a natural buster for body heat. They smeared mud all over their skins in order to tolerate their year-round hot and humid climate. The famous *din so porng* (white mud) is Thailand's traditional answer to an SPF. Its alkaline balance cools down the skin and replenishes moisture to prevent sun damage and subsequent skin disease.

However, like many of tropical Asia's natural remedies, *din so porng*, turns out to be an all-body panacea: it prevents perspiration, reduces fever, heals wounds, clears rashes and retains the skin's healthy, natural glow, as well as acting as an all-over cooler.

The mud, with its gypsum mineral content, can be applied in its natural state. But being the alchemists they are, Thai people commonly mix *din so porng* into scented balls with pollen and bark which they smoke in a fragrant talcum powder. These are simply crushed and applied for the ultimate skin food. Alternatively they can be combined with some specific perfumes for scented skin, or used as a body scrub to combat skin disease — even repair puss-infested wounds!

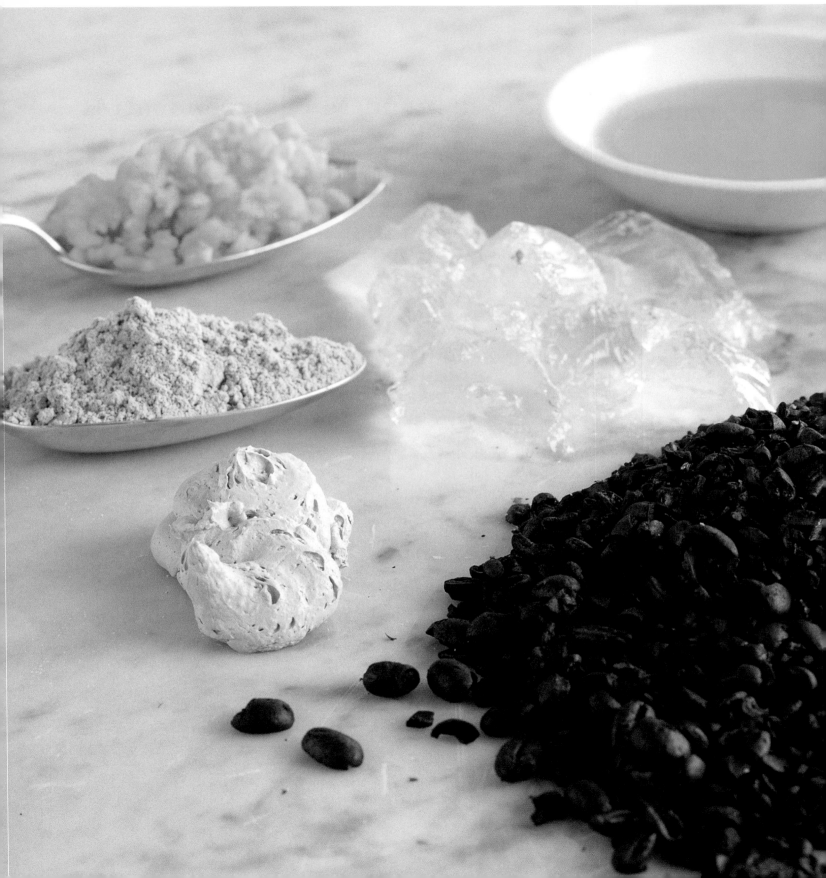

Bali Kopi Scrub

If you swoon when you pass a city coffee bar, imagine *that* smell for a full 45 minutes while the most fragrant of blends is smothered all over your body. Admittedly this coffee body scrub was only recently invented to cater for our addiction to the aroma of freshly ground beans. In Indonesia, where this scrub is offered, people stick to drinking the stuff, less as an excuse to sit and chat and more to give them energy while they work.

This scrub, rougher than some and ideal for male skin, is offered at all Mandara Spas (at *The Chedi, Ibah, Bali Padma* and *Nikko* in Bali), the *Novotel* in Lombok and Malaysia's *The Datai*) according to this recipe.

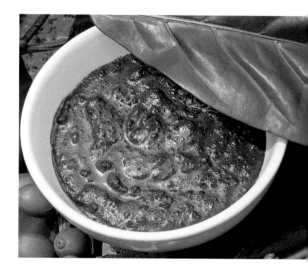

Ingredients

200 gms (6 oz)	Balinese coffee beans, ground
40 gms (3 tbsp)	kaolin clay (or cosmetic clay available at health shops)
pinch	ground pumice stone (optional)
1/4 kilo (1/2 lb)	carrots, grated or blended
10 gms (1 tsp)	gelatin, already set (optional)

Steps

1 Balinese coffee is the most fragrant of all Indonesian varieties, but you can substitute this for your favourite blend. Crush the dried beans quite finely and mix with the kaolin clay and ground pumice. Add a splash of water.

2 Rub over the entire body, later rubbing more vigorously so that the mixture sloughs off.

3 Rub the carrot, which can be mixed with the gelatin for easier application, into your body to replenish any lost moisture during the exfoliation process.

4 Shower and moisturize.

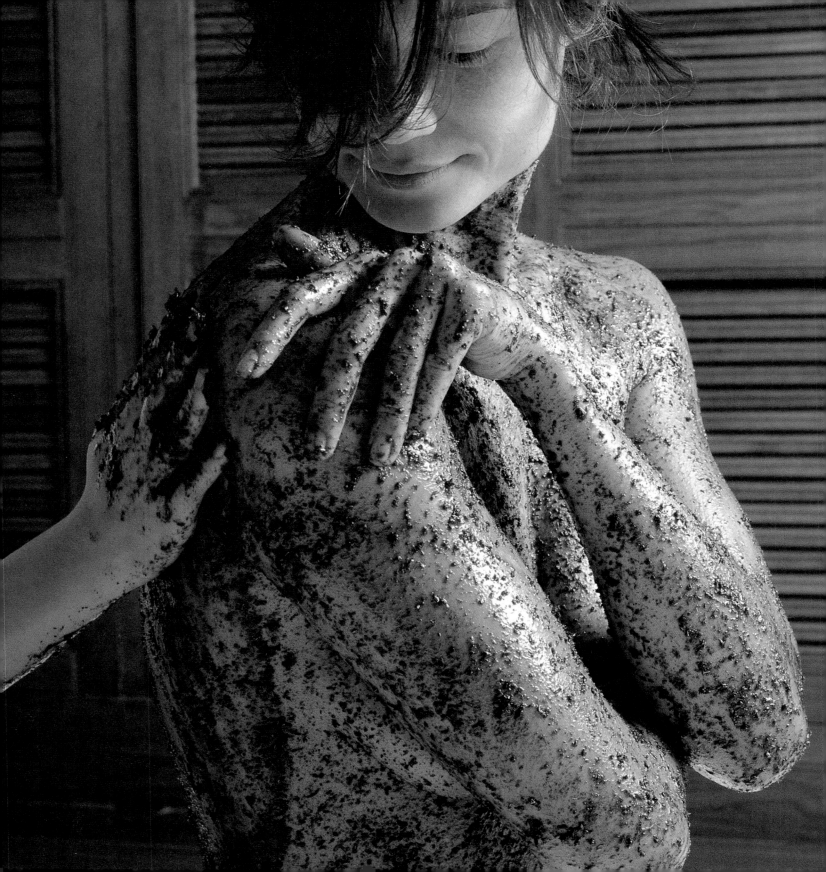

Oriental Body Glow

For the invigorating rather than relaxing route to soft skin, this traditional Thai body scrub is the way forward. It is on the menu at the *The Oriental Spa*, Bangkok and the *Banyan Tree Spa Phuket*.

Ingredients

1 cup	runny honey
¹/₂ cup	sesame seeds
sprinkling	dried herbs: lavender leaf, mint (which makes the mixture turn dark)

Steps

1 Mix the ingredients together and rub the thick, sticky paste over your body. Take your time so that the skin properly exfoliates and make the most of the sweet aroma reminiscent of that childhood smell of cooking caramel.

2 Shower. The whole process takes about half an hour.

Honey Treats

The humectant properties of honey nourish and moisturize the skin. You can use honey on both face and body. In Thailand, where it is produced under royal patronage in the north of the country, honey has traditionally been used to cover open wounds in order to soften scar tissue and encourage the growth of new skin.

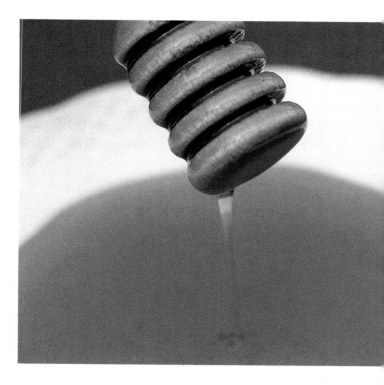

Face

1 Massage runny honey – with a squeeze of lime for astringent purposes or some ground oatmeal if you like a coarser texture – into damp skin for 15 minutes.

2 Rinse your face with warm water to leave it feeling soft and peeled.

Body

1 Cover body with honey and sit in the steam room.

2 Shower.

Such a gentle treatment can be used two or three times a week for normal to dry skin.

Thai Herbal Heat Revival

This heated muslin parcel of aromatic herbs and spices is a heavenly health treatment in the raw; it is unchanged since Thailand's Ayutthaya period (14th –18th century) when a fragrant hot-pack was administered to war-weary soldiers returning home with muscle aches and bruises.

Today the poultice is still used to alleviate pain or inflammation (especially good post partum) by opening the pores and bringing a medicinal heat to the muscles to induce relaxation.

The Thai herbal pack is excellent at *The Oriental Spa*, Bangkok and *Banyan Tree Spa Phuket*. For an authentic steamy session, to soothe sore muscles and relax, combine the herb pack with a massage at the Thai Massage School, located in the corner of the beautiful Wat Po temple in Bangkok. Watch out for some real heat here and some temporary yellow skin staining (from the turmeric), but leave feeling better than believed possible!

Fill the parcel with a random mixture of the following straight from the kitchen of *The Oriental Spa*, Bangkok:

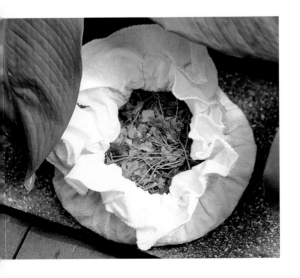

Ingredients
prai (common Thai herb)	for relief of sore muscles and tired joints
turmeric	an anti-bacterial skin freshener
lemon grass	an astringent for skin blemishes
Kaffir lime	for toning mature skin and for boosting circulation
camphor	for cleansing minor infections

Steps
1 Packed tight the parcel should be pomelo size, weighing roughly 400 gms (³/₄ lb).
2 The pack should be heated over a steamer or hot pot. It can be left steaming until needed, at least five minutes.
3 The poultice can be placed anywhere on the body for 30 seconds to one minute in each place. It should not be used on the face or genital area. It is good for slimming.

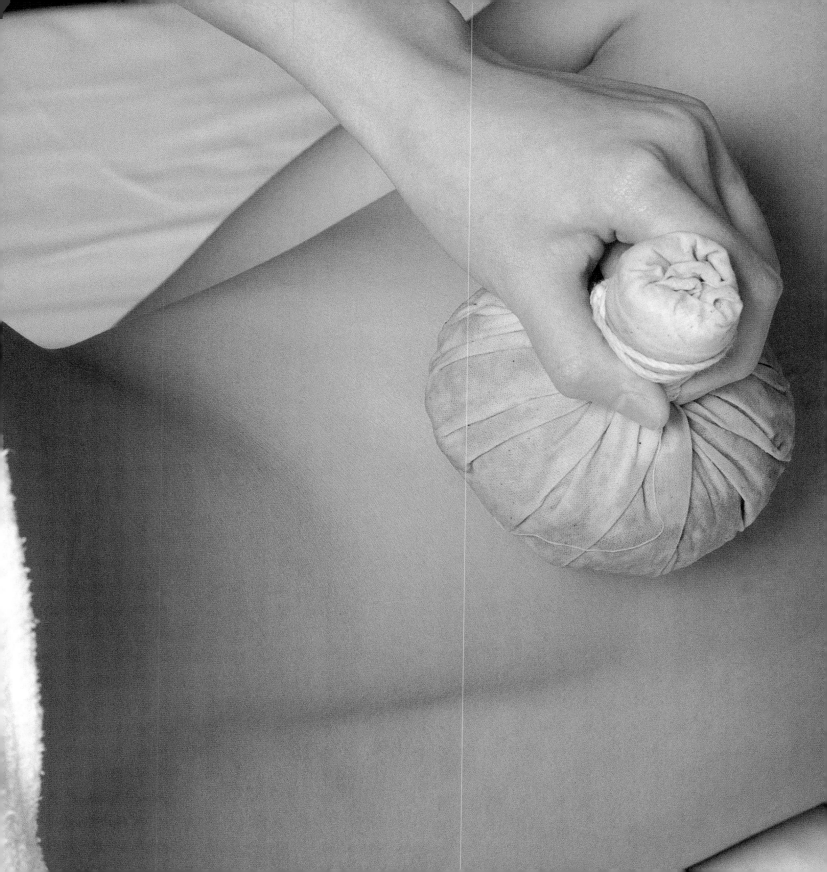

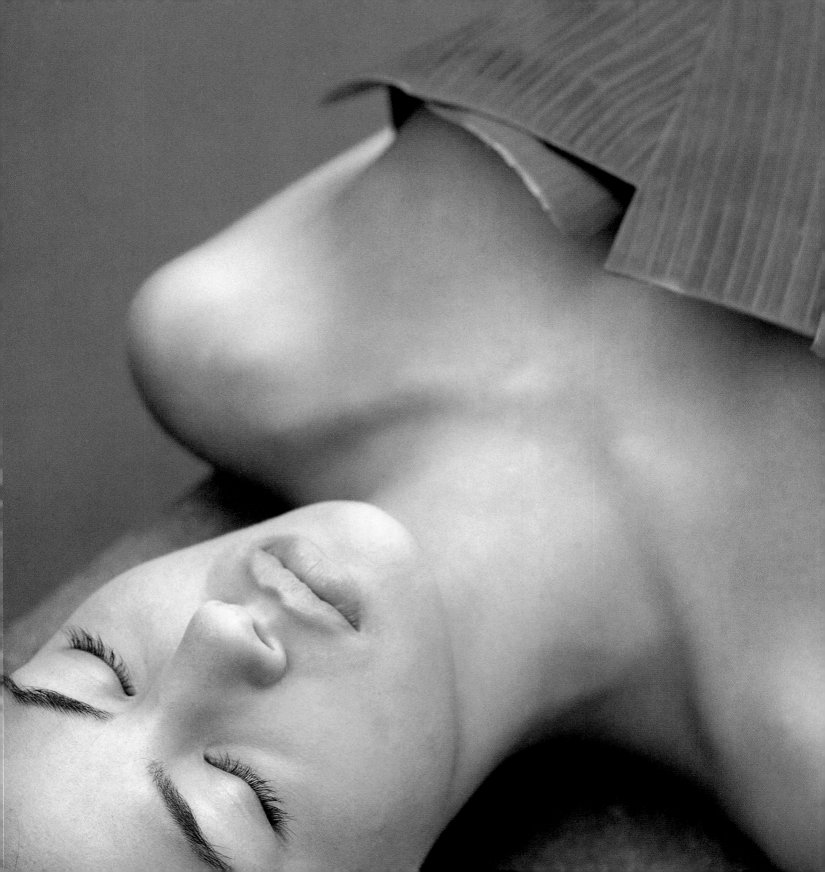

Aloe and Lavender Wrap

Aloe is grown and used in abundance in Indonesia, its long, spiny leaves cut and squeezed to release a sticky juice, ideal to pacify upset skin, stimulate the scalp and add fullness and lustre to hair.

While aloe is a major ingredient in all kinds of sensitive skin products, there is nothing more seductive than a coating of aloe, lavender and banana leaves, offered in this wrap at the *Spa at Jimbaran,* Four Seasons Resort Bali.

Ingredients

1 tsp	fresh aloe
to cover body	aloe vera gel (store bought)
a few spritzes	lavender essential oil mixed with distilled water
12 pieces	banana leaves (approximately 20 cm x 10 cm)
4	lemons or limes, cut in half
few drops	lavender essential oil
generous amount	lavender body lotion (or your favourite)

Steps

1   Stir the fresh aloe into the bought aloe gel and smear the mixture over the body, but first rub it between your palms to take off the chill. With a good gel, this feels wonderfully soft and slippery, rather than sticky on the skin.

2   Spritz the lavender essential oil in distilled water over your body for a heady fragrance.

3   Place the banana leaf patches over the top of your body and round your arms, so that all limbs are loosely covered. According to Balinese tradition you should not lie on top of banana leaves as this denotes part of the ritual that prepares a body for cremation. While banana leaves are not beneficial to the skin in themselves, they do help to take the heat from the body. They feel gentle and soothing on the skin without feeling cold. A cotton sarong can be placed on top to keep the leaves in position. Lie still for 20 minutes.

4   As the wrap is conditioning and relaxing the skin, this is the ideal moment for a head massage from a friend or loved one!

5   Remove leaves and shower; then douse your body with warm water infused with the juice of the lemons or limes and a few drops of lavender essential oil. Together these rinse and soothe the skin.

6   Finish with lavender body lotion.

Java Wrap

The Java Wrap is a global beauty phenomenon waiting to happen: an age-old process for a new-age answer to slimming. It started out as a 40-day ritual to rid the midriff from post birth bagginess and, even today, the Indonesian woman lovingly restores her body this way. It is believed that the Java Wrap helps flush out the bacteria which gather in the body after childbirth. It gets the lymphatic system going, reawakens the body's organs, and cleanses and heals.

New mothers can also benefit from the mineral and citrus paste that is smeared around the middle, then bound tight in a cotton corset. As the old saying goes: "you have to suffer for beauty". This figure-saving treatment is time-consuming rather than really uncomfortable, unless you visit the *St Gregory Javana Spa* in Singapore where all the work is done for you.

The special paste recipe is fairly standard throughout Indonesia where it has been handed down from one generation to another, and administered woman to woman in the household. This treatment is best done by one friend to another.

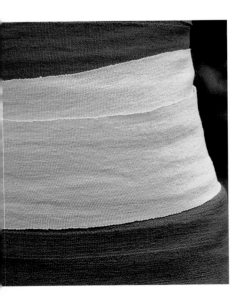

Ingredients

eucalyptus	strong antiseptic, benefits digestion
crushed sea stone/coral	calcium and other mineral content which warms and firms
fresh lime juice	an astringent which flushes toxins from the body
betel leaf	a leaf with antiseptic properties to cleanse womanly odour
massage oil	containing mint and eucalyptus essential oils for anti-viral and decongestant properties, also cooling.
cotton cummerbund	8–10 m long, 10–20 cm wide (8–10 yds long, 1 ft wide)

Steps

1. Mix enough ingredients to half-fill a cereal bowl with sufficient massage oil to give the paste a tacky texture that sticks to the body.
2. Rub the paste gently from above the tummy button to below the bottom.
3. Let it dry for 10 minutes, so that its healing properties start to soak into the skin.
4. Wrap the cummerbund neatly and tightly around the body starting under the bottom and weaving upward to the waist. The wrap physically constricts the body and helps to squeeze it back into shape!
5. Leave for 20 minutes, shower and moisturize with a gentle oil or lotion.
6. Post partum women in Indonesia also drink copious amounts of nourishing tonics such as turmeric, lime or betel leaf water.

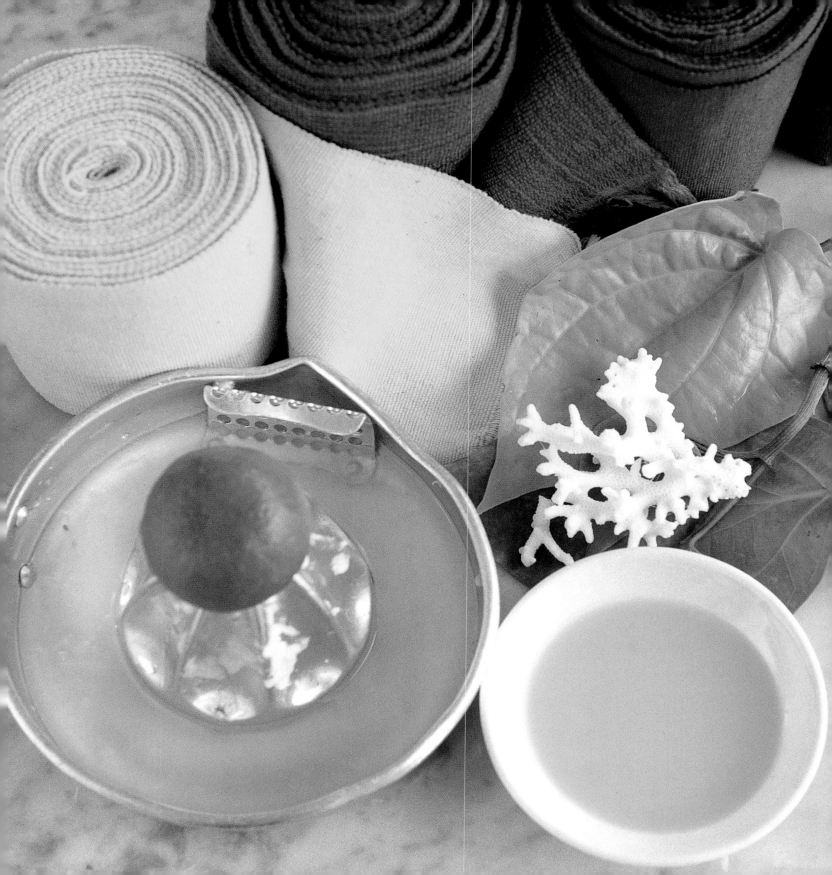

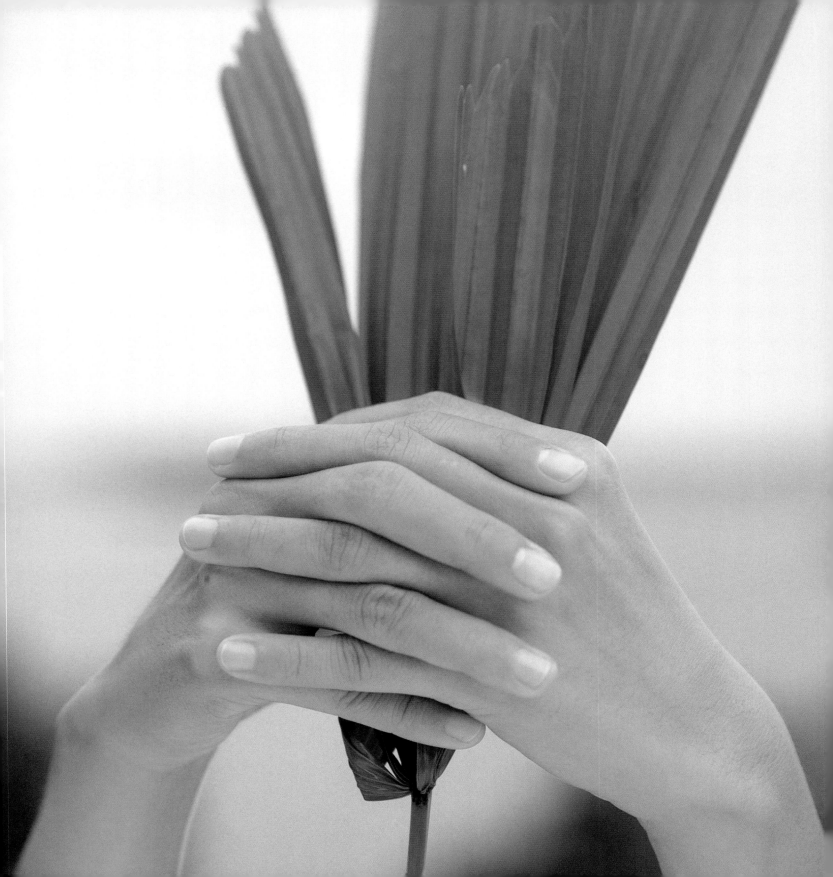

rites of massage

The power of touch is part of being human; it is part of our earliest awareness of being alive as babies in our mothers' arms. However, most people live in cultures that leave them isolated from one another. They give themselves no time to enjoy the simple pleasures of physical contact unless confined to the intimacy of the bedroom.

This is not the case in tropical Asia where massage is a part of everyday life from birth. Asian people understand that massage is all about sensual healing for the emotions as well as for the body, a simple and effective route to general wellbeing via our largest sensory organ – our skin. Skin is equipped with thousands of touch receptors; reacting to external stimuli, they transmit messages and sensations through our nervous system.

Massage is probably the oldest and simplest form of health care. It is depicted in Egyptian tomb paintings and mentioned in ancient Chinese, Japanese and Indian texts. It is thought to have originated in the East as a method for unblocking the *chi*, the vital energy flowing through our bodies that tends to get trapped due to emotional and physical upset. In Asia, massage has always been the backbone of health and wellbeing.

There is no mystery to the power of massage. The uncomplicated process of kneading, stroking and pressing the body is proven to unleash countless therapeutic benefits from the general: helping heart rate, blood pressure, breathing and digestion, to the more specific: aiding diabetic children, premature babies and cancer and HIV patients.

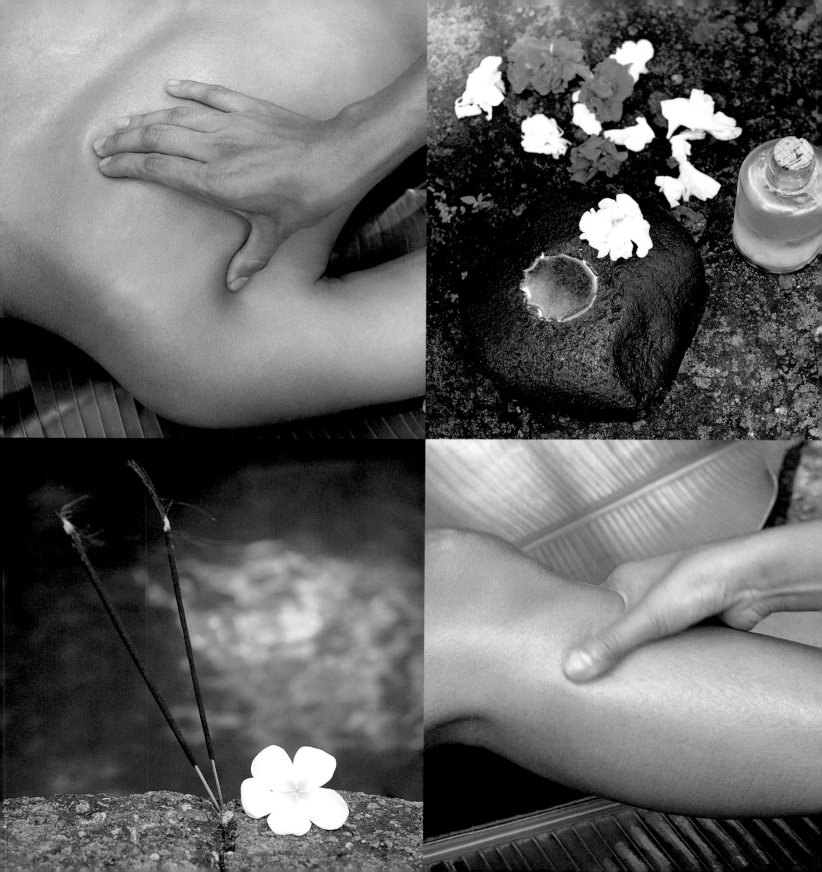

Traditional Indonesian Massage

We are creatures designed for touch. It is certainly the most personally experienced of all sensations. And the Indonesian people understand this better than most. Low-touch Western society keeps tactile expression behind closed doors, while Indonesians touch all the time: walking hand in hand and arm in arm, and stroking each other as a way of life.

They carry compassion in their hands. This they pass on naturally through massage to all the family from birth to death. Without a working knowledge of anatomy, many Indonesian people have an in-built sensibility to congested, tight or hot areas in the body, which they carefully relieve with the power of their hands and the application of aromatic oils.

It's interesting that Western culture, that has put so much faith in science for cures, and in medical practitioners for answers, is now turning, disillusioned, to touch therapies: Reiki, kineisiology, cranial osteopathy, aromatherapy, reflexology, all variations on a cure practised for centuries by Asian peoples.

Indonesian massage puts touch back into your system. As well as an unconditional desire to please and an intuitive reaction to the body, here is what to expect:

- medium pressure.
- scented massage oil: coconut oil prepared with local flowers such as champak (tropical magnolia), *akar wangi* (vetiver) and pandanus leaf is the traditional preparation; however, coconut is a heavy oil not suited to everyone, and is not always used in spas. (Balinese people chew on the white flesh, ingest the juices, spit out the fibres and rub them onto their skins for nourishment).
- long sensual strokes, working the length of the muscle to relieve tension. All sequences finish with upward strokes toward the heart.
- rolling skin between thumb and forefinger to spark up the nerve endings and increase blood flow.
- circular thumb movements for the same.
- pressure on the points in the foot and hand reflex zones.

Carrier Oils

Essential oils are too strong to be applied neat to the skin so when used in massage they should be mixed with a carrier or base oil, usually a cold pressed vegetable oil which has its own beneficial properties.

To obtain the correct proportions for a massage blend, add a number of drops of essential oil equivalent to half the number of millilitres of carrier oil. For example, for an average body size, pour 10 mls of carrier oil (or combination) into a bowl that is not plastic and add five drops of essential oil (or a combination of up to three oils).

Store massage blends in blue or amber glass away from sunlight to keep essential oils fresh. Vegetable oils should be used within 6–8 months before they turn rancid. Otherwise blend them with wheatgerm. Here are some of the oils most commonly used in an Asian tropical spa:

Almond

This vaguely aromatic oil is gentle and rich in proteins and vitamins. It is nourishing, light and softening for dry hands, eczema and irritated skin. It is a good lubricant, so blends well with other oils as an excellent massage base.

Avocado

This is a rich, heavy oil with high vitamin content. It is often blended for a velvet-like consistency. It also contains a mild sunscreen.

Coconut

Traditionally, this was the main carrier oil in tropical Asia because of its abundance. It is a thick saturated oil with its own distinct smell. It remains stable for a long period and is particularly nourishing in hair treatments.

Grapeseed

This is an extremely fine and pure oil, so light it absorbs immediately into the skin. It is good for helping the essential oils penetrate quickly. It leaves a satiny, not sticky, coating.

Jojoba

This is a natural fluid wax rather than an oil. It has a fine consistency (similar to collagen) which effectively penetrates the skin. It reputedly nourishes hair and prevents hair loss.

Macadamia

The acids in this oil are natural components of skin sebum. It has a rich nutty aroma and consistency. Its emollient qualities make it a good all round moisturizer, particularly for dry and mature skin.

Olive

Rich in proteins and vitamins, this oil is rapidly absorbed by the skin although it has a strong aroma and is often blended with other oils. It is a naturally warming oil, so it is good for massage in cold weather or in treatments for muscular pains.

Wheatgerm

This is a rich, dark oil, high in vitamin E but sometimes thought too heavy and aromatic to use alone. It is an antioxidant: it stabilizes essential oils and other carrier oils, making them last longer. It also benefits scarring.

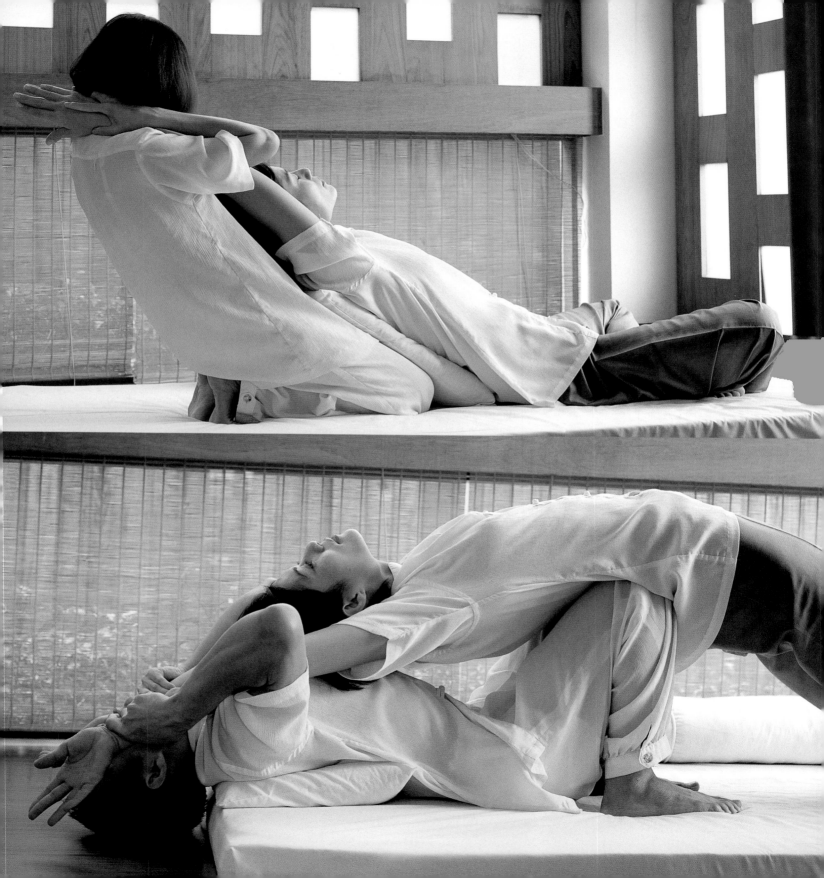

Thai Massage

It's the absence of oil and the addition of pyjamas that distinguishes Thai massage from all other massage therapies. Thai people claim that their skin is never dry enough, due to their country's hot climate, to need lubrication. They do, however, cover their bodies out of a sense of decorum in the face of some rather contorted positions! It is one of the ancient healing arts of traditional Thai medicine, the others being herbal medicine and spiritual meditation. Its style developed during the period of King Rama II out of the stretching techniques of Indian Ayurveda and the traditional Chinese focus on the body's pressure points. As a result, experts claim that Thai massage works more deeply than the more surface-oriented Swedish technique. It has an ability to heal, relax and realign the body.

By pressing on the body's energy meridians as well as its veins and muscle tips, Thai massage releases the sluggish flow of blood and build-up of toxins that gather in tired or overworked muscles. In a sense, it invigorates and heals them with a physical workout. This is combined with a spectacular technique, which mindfully stretches the limbs into positions that the uninitiated could never believe possible. Close body contact allows the masseur to hold, for example, the ankle in two hands, easing it away from the hips while pressing deep with his foot into muscles in the inner thigh. Such postures stretch the tendons and ligaments while making the body more supple, realigning it and releasing tension.

If this sounds more acrobatic than agreeable, be assured that good Thai masseurs, immersed in the 'middle way' of Buddhism, take a calm, meditative (not just physical) approach to their work, sensing the energy patterns in a person's body. Skilled therapists always start by softly squeezing the limbs with the palm of their hands in order to warm up the body and listen to its needs.

Important Body Parts in Thai Massage

Feet
Masseurs always start with the feet as this is where the whole body weight rests. Awakening the reflex points prepares the rest of the body for the massage.

Scalp
While nothing penetrates beneath the skull, massage along the scalp lines increases blood flow to the head where much of the body's tension is stored.

Ears
Masseurs spend a lot of time stretching and pulling these reflexology sensors, releasing headaches and helping with balance.

Face
A gentle fingertip pressure, Thai style, will release tension to increase blood flow and prevent wrinkles, while excessive pummeling will create them.

Essential Oils

The following essential oils are traditional to Southeast Asia. Best quality oils are extracted from plants (usually the leaves, flowers, roots or berries) through a process of steam distillation. As French aromatherapist Danielle Ryman points out: "extraction is a painstaking process as the amount of oil present in plants is minute."

Before the process of distillation, which has remained virtually unchanged for hundreds of years, people used medicinal plants in their lives by eating them, rubbing them onto wounds or making them into teas, poultices, tinctures and ointments.

Plants, flowers and their essences have played an integral role in healing disciplines in Asia and the rest of the world for thousands of years. 'Aromatherapy', as we know it today – the art and science of treating illness and emotions with essential oils – was formalized by a French chemist, Dr R M Gattefosse in the early 20th century.

The powerful properties of essential oils are best absorbed through the skin or through inhalation. Their aroma can eliminate blocks and restore body balance. They are great companions for the emotions they can ignite and help they can bring in promoting health and harmony in our modern lifestyles.

Clove

• This small evergreen tree originates from the coasts of the Moluccas in Indonesia but is now grown in most tropical climes. Its flowering buds turn into the familiar brown cloves when dried and these, along with the leaves, are distilled into the oil.
• A strong, woody base note with a sweet, spicy vanilla scent.
• Clove oil is an antiseptic and anaesthetic: a drop on a sore tooth will numb the ache. It is a general tonic for physical and intellectual weakness and is known to help overcome frigidity, claiming similar properties to opium. It is valued for its digestive properties, so when massaged into the abdomen, it relieves pain and diarrhea. Suck a clove if you are feeling stressed or wish to give up smoking. Infused into the atmosphere, clove will brighten the spirits.

Ginger

• The oil is distilled from the tuberous, pungent root of the tropical plant which originated in India but is now grown in many countries.
• A warm and spicy fragrance with a stimulating, almost lemon top note.
• Ginger is well known for its aphrodisiac qualities best administered by mixing with a base oil for massage in the lower spine. It eases muscular aches and pains and is therefore good for menstrual cramps. It relieves flu symptoms and its warming qualities help sweat out fevers and colds and treat digestive disorders.

Jasmine

• The fragrant white jasmine blossoms come from an evergreen shrub grown all over Asia. Jasmine symbolizes the sweetness of a woman and is the flower most used in perfumery: it reputedly takes more than 10,000 crushed heads to produce one ounce of *Joy*, Jean Patou's famous fragrance and one of the most expensive in the world.
• The aroma is sweet and euphoric.
• Jasmine uplifts the soul; it is used as a sign of friendship and as a Buddhist offering in Thailand. Indonesian women weave the flowers into newly washed and oiled hair to infuse it with perfume. It relieves pre-menstrual mood swings and pains as well as labour pains when applied as a compress. It softens dry skin and reduces stretch marks. It unearths compassion and inspires artistic creativity. Use the oil in a burner, in massage, or in the bath to feel seductive.

Nutmeg

• A sturdy evergreen tree that originated in the Spice Islands. The kernels of the fruits are the nutmeg, while its red lacy covering is mace. In cookery, it is used in cakes and curries.
• Warm and spicy with musky overtones.
• Nutmeg aids the digestive system by breaking down starches and fats. Used sparingly in massage oils, its warmth helps muscular aches and pains and stimulates the circulation. It is especially good to strengthen contractions in childbirth, and also has purifying properties.

Patchouli

• While patchouli is native to Malaysia, 450 of the 550-tonne annual world production comes out of Sumatra, Indonesia, from a small, fragrant shrub bearing white flowers, tinged purple.
• Strong, woody, wet and earthy fragrance.
• In the West, patchouli oil was favoured by the flower children of the 1960s for its flair for arousing sexual passion and psychic awareness. In the East, this oil is redolent of Bali where it is burned everywhere to create a relaxing atmosphere. Patchouli is great for skin conditions, mixed with oil for acne, eczema, burns and scar tissue.

Sandalwood

• The best sandalwood comes from plantations in Mysore, India. The oil is extracted from the roots and the centre of the slender trunk when the sandalwood tree is 50 years old.
• Syrupy, sweet, thick and heady aroma.
• Of all aromatics, sandalwood plays the supreme role in eastern religious ceremony, symbolizing spirituality. It is a major cosmetic ingredient, particularly in oriental perfume. Use it in massage oil to treat dry skin, in baths to relieve cystitis and infections, and in burners to calm the nervous system and promote clarity of thought. This is a particularly grounding and balancing oil.

Vetiver

• Vetiver oil comes from the roots of vetiver grass grown largely in India and Indonesia.
• Deep smoky base note, with a woody yet sweetly spicy undertone.
• Known as the 'oil of tranquillity' in India for its deeply relaxing effect, vetiver is traditionally woven into mats or screens and hung in rooms to evoke a sedative atmosphere. It keeps insects away, and while it stimulates blood flow and relieves muscle tension, it also stimulates the production of breast milk if massaged with oil into the chest. Like sandalwood, it is beneficial for anxiety as well as insomnia and helps you cope in times of upheaval.

Ylang-Ylang

• The ylang-ylang tree is known as the 'crown of the east' and the 'perfume tree' due to the overwhelmingly sweet smell of its flowers. It originated in the Philippines and is grown all over tropical Asia.
• Sumptuous and sugary fragrance with high notes like hyacinth and narcissus.
• In Indonesia the beds of newlyweds are scattered with ylang-ylang to proffer luck, harmony and fertility. Indeed, the oil is a famed aphrodisiac, most effective when dropped into bath water. By stirring the emotions, ylang-ylang resolves conflicts between partners and brings harmony, peace and warmth. It is good for nervous, stressed people and is an effective skin treatment and sun tanning aid when mixed with nut oils.

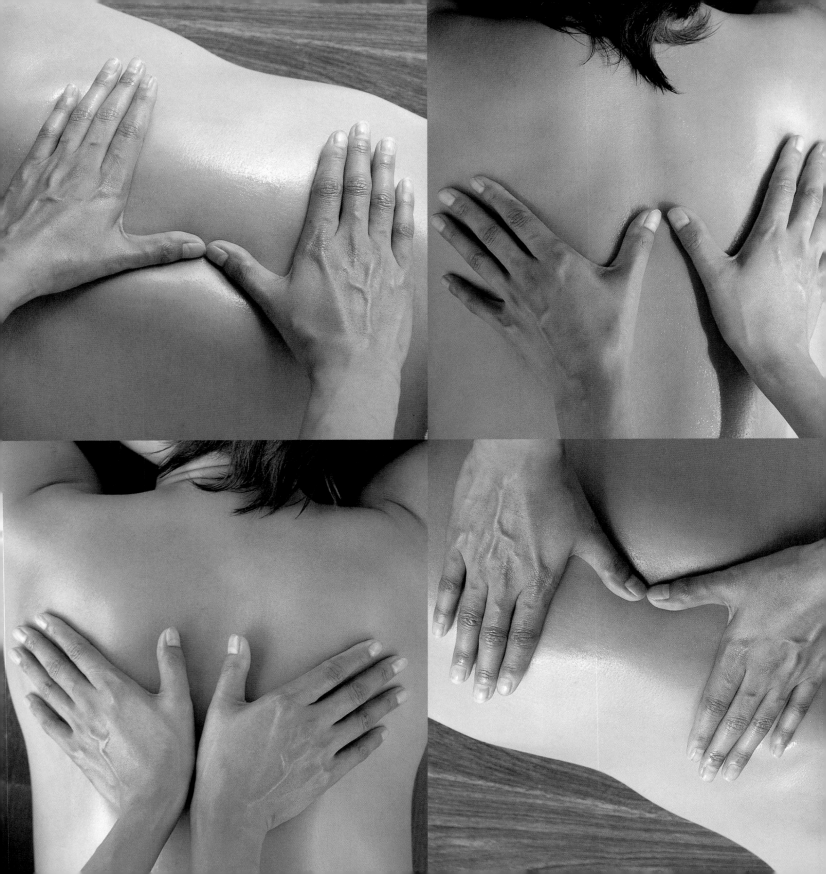

Aromatherapy Massage

Aromatherapy massage is one of the most popular treatments at a tropical spa. Although available throughout the world, its sensual experience is elevated to new levels in Asia thanks to the gentle and sensitive nature of its practitioners. Therapists appear to approach each and every massage as a bespoke, individual craft, rather than another body on their daily production line.

Through massage the active molecules of essential oils, already blended with a carrier oil, penetrate the bloodstream and soothe the central nervous system. For most people, the barrage of citrus, floral or spicy notes of the oils, like any smell, will bring back a stream of memories. The physiology of smell and emotion are supposedly closely linked. Apparently the olfactory sensors in our nasal passage can recognize up to 10,000 different aromas. In addition, as the massage activates the body's nerve endings and stimulates its blood flow, the medicinal properties of essential oils act on the internal organs and treat ailments. Although the oils only remain in the body for three or four hours before they are excreted, they have already triggered a healing process.

Mandara Massage

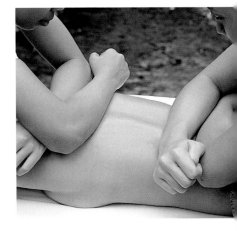

The Mandara Massage is the zenith of massage experience. This is thanks to the uncanny sychronization of two therapists who work together all over the body. The melodic rhythm of their strokes creates a pattern of sensation so pleasurable that you feel almost guilty for the indulgence. With one at the top and one at the toe, the therapists' hands move in harmony with each other, without ever leaving your skin. Their unique combination of six massage styles: Hawaiian Lomi-Lomi, Swedish, Balinese, Japanese Shiatsu, Thai and Aromatherapy ensures that every nerve ending is caressed. This is hypnotic, exotic and euphoric.

The Mandara Massage was exclusively devised for Mandara Spas (at *The Chedi, Ibah, Bali Padma* and *Nikko* in Bali, *Novotel* in Lombok and Malaysia's *The Datai*). It takes its name from the Mandara of Balinese legend – a mythical mountain that flows with eternal youth. Translated into an earthly equivalent, this massage is as close as one gets to such a sublime concept.

Tropical Oil Blends

Blending essential oils is an enriching part of aromatherapy. It opens up a Pandora's Box of fragrant opportunities. By composing your own blend you can strike the perfect note for your mood and discover your own way to sensual healing.

Many tropical spas and natural product companies have come up with their own scented oil blends to enhance the seductive nature of the various treatments for body, mind and soul. Here are some of the most inviting:

Peace of Bali Oil

Exclusive to the *Spa at Jimbaran*, Four Seasons Resort, this oil is a sacred blend of sandalwood, ylang-ylang and a touch of citrus. The combination has a calming and grounding effect just like the natural peace that Bali bestows.

Bali Sunset Oil

A splash of nutmeg essential oil adds warmth to any massage blend. This oil from the *Spa at Jimbaran*, Four Seasons Resort, focuses on nutmeg, with a touch of vetiver and lemon grass. It is used as a symbol of the warmth of the sun and the radiant sunset which is magnificent at this spot on the island's coast.

Bali Santi

Prepared according to traditional methods in Ubud, Bali, this oil from *Utama Spice* is a rich blend of coconut oil infused with vetiver, patchouli and other herbs for pure relaxation.

Java Oil

By *Esens*, this is a stimulating blend of eucalyptus and peppermint, traditionally used as an analgesic as well as a headache remedy. It is a good blend to use when slimming.

Bali Oil

From *Esens* comes a wonderful all-round blend named simply, redolent of the romance of the island where it was born. A coconut oil base is infused with pandanus leaf, champak flowers and vetiver according to an old village recipe for body and hair.

The *Scents and Elixirs* range of oil blends from *Essential* is used at *Nusa Dua Spa*:

Exotic Fruits

A blend of citrus essential oils for uplifting the spirit. It is redolent of the fruits and flowers that are seen everywhere in Bali on the myriad offerings to the Gods.

Sensual Flowers

This blend, dominated by the floral ylang-ylang oil, is reminiscent of Bali's many ceremonies and the abundant flowers they include. The significance of nature is so powerful for the Balinese that they believe the sweeter the flower the quicker their prayer will rise to heaven.

Desert Spice

A curative blend, heavy with ginger essential oil, warms the body and embraces the mood of the Spice Islands. Varieties of this oil have been used for centuries during the rainy season.

Oils enjoyed at *Mandara Spas* include:

Mandara Oil

The signature blend from *Mandara Spas* is an oil for romance. Its main ingredients are sandalwood and patchouli and it is also recommended for dry and scaly skin conditions.

Harmony Oil

Which speaks for itself. The blend of citrus fruits, canaga and other floral essences balance the body, mind and spirit.

Tranquillity Oil

A relaxing blend of vetiver, ylang-ylang and other calming essential oils that relax and warm the body.

Bali Santai Oil

A rejuvenating and gentle oil concentrated with mandarin essential oil, especially soothing for a pregnant mother.

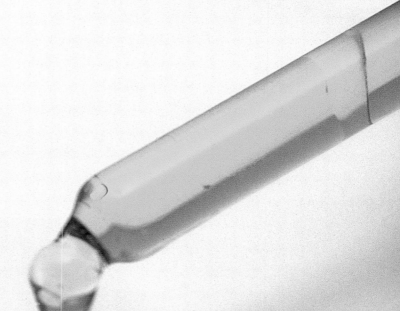

Rich and highly fragrant jojoba oil blends used at the *Spa at Bali Hyatt* include:

Stargaze Body Oil

Mixes cedarwood for stress reduction and a whiff of rose and orange to refresh and uplift.

Spirit Body Oil

Re-energizing oil that blends grapefruit for cell regeneration, lemon grass for muscle purification and lavender to calm the nerves so that you rise feeling recharged.

Sunset Body Oil

Best applied as an after-sun, thanks to the anti-inflammatory German camomile which soothes irritation. Together with sandalwood and lavender it has a sedating effect.

Moonlight Body Oil

Helps to gain balance in the body and stimulate cell growth if the skin has been sunburnt. This oil is a blend of frankincense which comforts, vetivert which has anti-inflammatory properties, sandalwood which strengthens the spirit and rose which is a balancing oil.

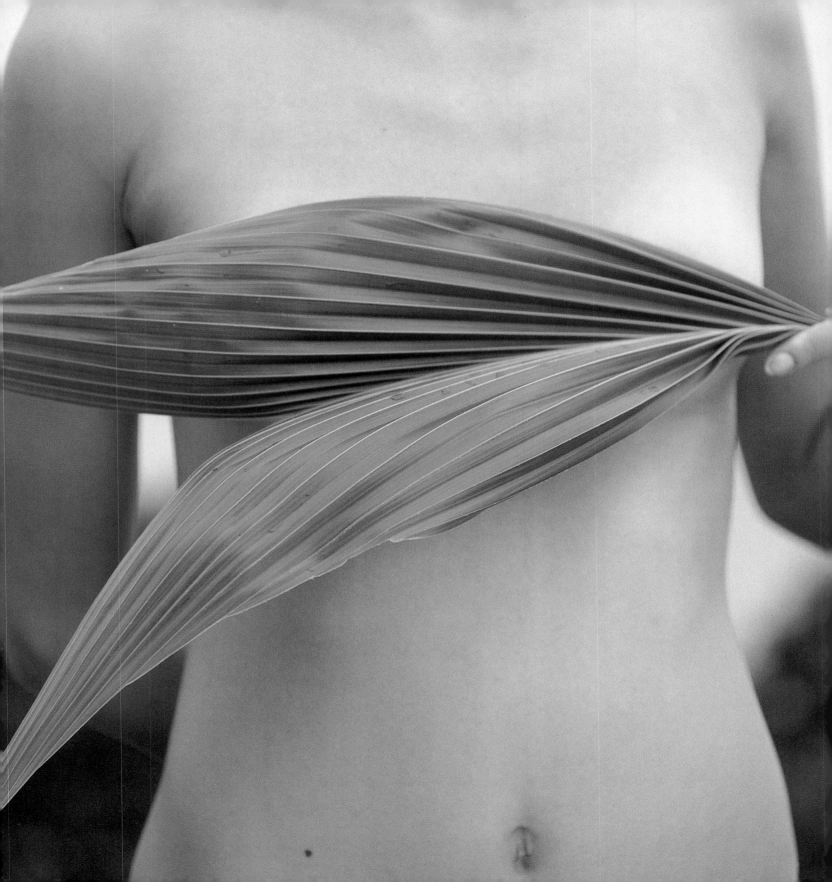

m i n d - b o d y - s p i r i t

There was a time, not so long ago, when the notion of beauty was literally skin deep. A costly cosmetic, where packaging was an artwork in itself, was the final answer to a smooth and clear complexion. It all ended here in the gold-topped tub.

Not any more. The materialistic '80s have given way to the caring '90s and a whole new approach to beauty that stems from within. It's the realization that it is not just our bodies but our minds and souls that need attention, if we are to be the radiant creatures that we all aspire to. Beauty no longer simply means a 'boob job' or a 'nose job', it means the pursuit of 'mindfulness', the latest buzz word for an overall sense of wellbeing that is deemed so important now.

In order to tap into this spiritual dimension, we are turning to mindful exercise – yoga, *tai chi*, meditation, even simple focused breathing techniques which offer physical and psychological benefits in one. All of this is a natural extension of the health and beauty treatments and the assault on all our senses which have come to represent the tropical spa philosophy. What is more: the mood for holistic self-preservation which has so recently become the favoured route to self-fulfilment in the West, has always been the unquestioned way of life in the East. Mindful exercise, in its varying guises, originated here in the simple belief that we can only look and feel good if our bodies and our spirits are working together in healthy harmony.

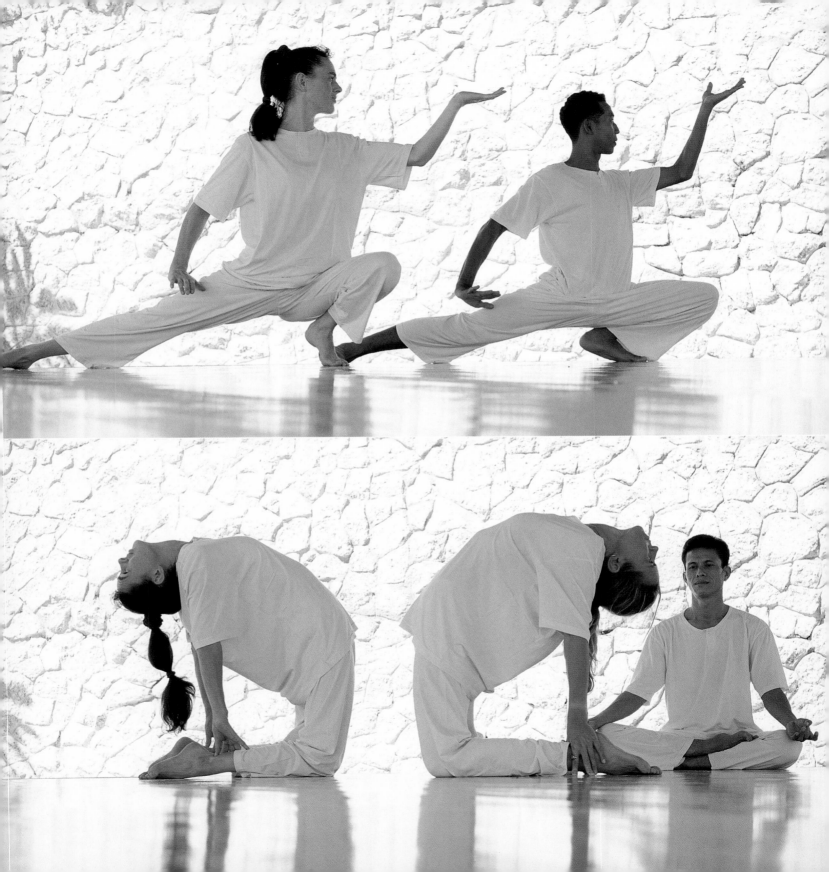

Tai Chi

This ancient Chinese movement therapy is all about harnessing the natural energy both within us and from outside. It relies on the belief that the smooth flow of *chi'* or life energy, through the body's meridians, is vital for good health and that illness occurs when there is an imbalance or sluggish flow in certain areas due to anxiety, tension and fatigue.

Tai chi is similar to yoga with its focus on breathing and its slow, meditative movements that concentrate our minds and encourage us to listen to that which we can never really hear: our inner self. However, *tai chi* has its own system of graceful arm movements that symbolize the deliberate process of harnessing the earth's energy and drawing it into our bodies. These movements, combined with strong leg postures, are learnt as a sequence practised time and again, although the sequence varies according to proficiency levels. Experts will practise the long version combining up to 108 movements in a 30-minute session.

Yoga

In its purest form yoga is a complete system of physical and mental training: a series of spiritual stages on the path to enlightenment dating back to 1200 BC in India when its wisdom and practice were passed down from Hindu ascetic guru to disciple.

The global spread of interest in yoga in the 20th century is unprecedented although much of its appeal lies in the catch-all benefits it unleashes: its ability to work on muscle groups, increase suppleness and vitality, tone internal organs, stimulate nerve centres, relieve stress and clear the mind. All this is attained through breathing techniques (*pranayama*) and physical postures (*asanas*) performed deliberately and slowly with a concentrated focus on our own inner awareness.

Yoga looks upon the body as the temple of the soul and in this respect is becoming a far more attractive alternative to the all-brawn-no-brain step class. Indeed exercise at its most seductive is a twilight yoga class under a Thai-style pavilion beside the beach at Thailand's *Chiva-Som* where the sea breezes and mantras help transport you to inner realms you never knew you possessed.

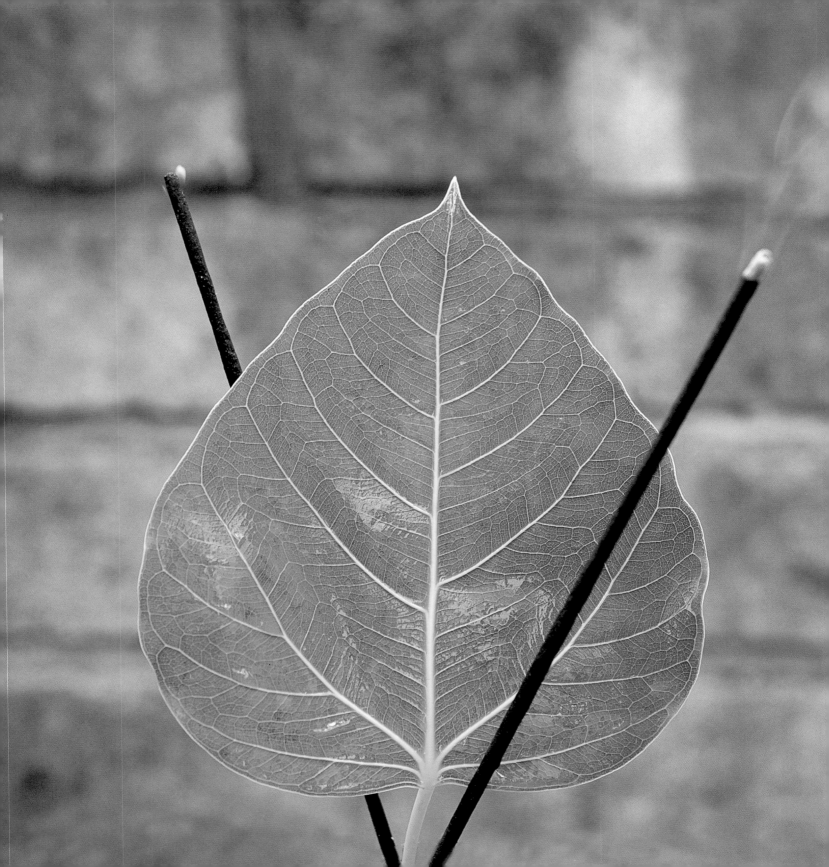

Meditation

It's all too easy to believe that meditation is a simple form of stress busting, that requires no physical workout and a bit of peace and quiet in which to breathe deeply and concentrate on 'nothing' in order to feel profoundly relaxed. For the uninitiated, this mental discipline is not so straightforward. It can be virtually impossible to drown out the incessant rabble of our internal dialogue and it takes practice to reach the state of heightened awareness and inner peace that meditation helps us to achieve.

The various techniques all involve focusing the mind on an object, colour or activity to which it can return if it gets distracted. These may include the conscious rhythm of breathing, a mantra – word or phrase such as 'Om', the most used and sacred mantra of the Hindus, or an icon such as a burning candle or religious statue.

Once in a quiet, receptive state, the mind excretes certain brain waves, known as alpha waves, that purportedly operate at a far higher intensity than those that occur during sleep, creating electrical activity that leads to altered awareness and deep relaxation.

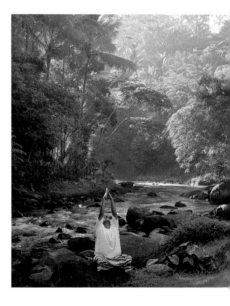

While different forms of meditation are practised in all major religions (in Christianity it takes the form of prayer), it is most readily associated with the spiritualism of the oriental world where it is used as a way of exploring the inner recesses of the mind and achieving a euphoric condition. This was picked up in the West during the 1960s when the Beatles popularized Transcendental Meditation (TM). By the 1990s, meditation in the West is no longer the preserve of the kaftan-clad fringe set, but has become an executive tool for beating stress, insomnia, addictions and depression.

It is best to be guided through the rudiments of meditation by a practitioner. However, some of the tranquil, tropical locations in Asia are so heavy with a spiritual silence that they provide a perfect sanctuary for getting started on the path to mindful relaxation. A location that immediately comes to mind is Sayan, outside Ubud in Bali, where sessions are offered at the *The Four Seasons* and *Begawan Giri Estate* by expert practitioners.

Yogaia Wave Movement

With so many forms of 'mindful' exercise currently in vogue, how do you choose what to focus on? Meditation clears the mind but doesn't do much for the cardiovascular and yoga is ideal as long as energy levels are not hitting the roof. This is where Yogaia Wave has found its niche. Called 'waving' by those in the know, this new exercise is a synthesis of forms that incorporates yoga, dance, martial arts positions and meditative practices, which together, bring a host of healing benefits. Who would have known that gyrating could do you so much good?

The co-founder of Yogaia Wave, Se'a Criss, is based at *Begawan Giri Estate*, Bali. She claims that this fun form of exercise realigns the body's physical structure, enhances the immune system, opens up the spinal column, balances the emotions and relieves anxiety – and, if this weren't enough – balances the left and right brain functions. Nevertheless, this is perfect for the 'mindful' exercise sceptic: it is a combination of aerobics without the schlep and yoga with a bit of pizzazz. In other words a complete mind and body workout.

Water Shiatsu Therapy

At last a grown up body treatment that makes us feel young again – really young. Water Shiatsu originated in America but has been developed as an aquatic body therapy for tropical waters by the *Breathing Space* in Singapore. It is so absorbing and comforting that it must – if only we could remember for sure – recreate the sensations of life in the womb. The rocking and gentle stretches, which are all part of this treatment, make you feel like a baby anyway!

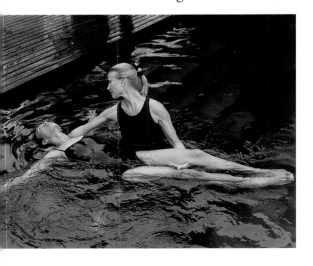

Thanks to the buoyancy of the water for support, the body relaxes in free float. This is the optimum state for carrying out bodywork according to the principles of shiatsu, the Japanese form of massage that concentrates on the body's meridians to stimulate its energy flow and de-stress. The mind goes into limbo as the body is walked very slowly around the pool and gently rocked. This is the starting point for various sequences that revolve, massage and outstretch the limbs. Ardent followers claim that the treatment helps them get in touch with deep feelings of safety and connectedness. However you choose to look at it, Water Shiatsu is – for sure – a total tune-out and the ultimate unwind! Try it at a *Breathing Space* weekend retreat or at their *Moana Spa*, both on the Indonesian island of Batam.

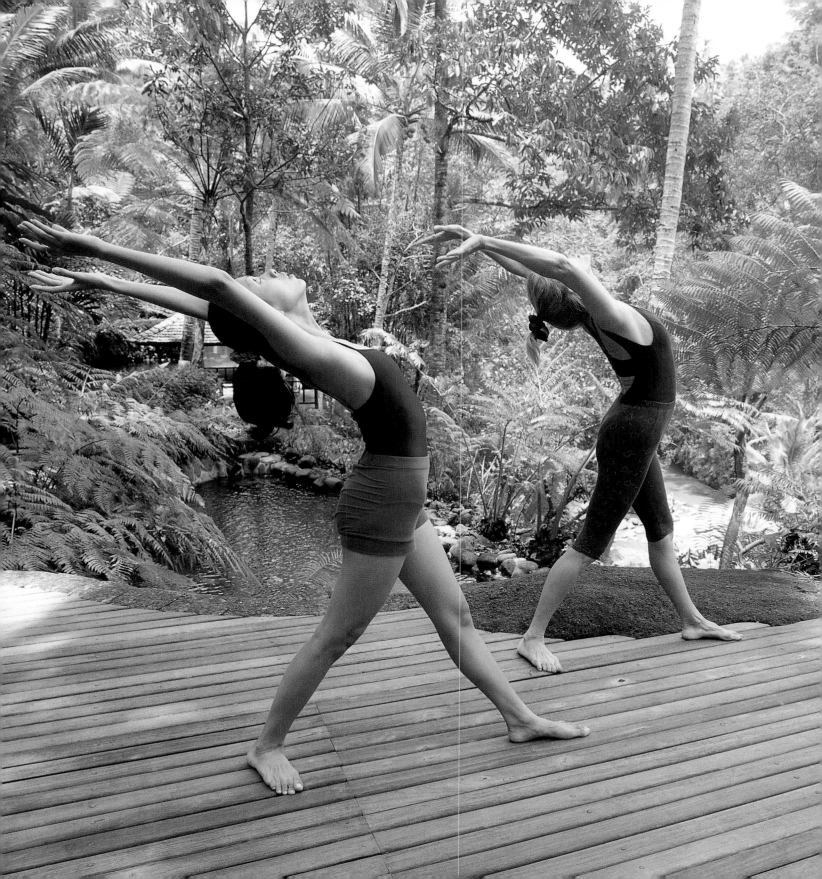

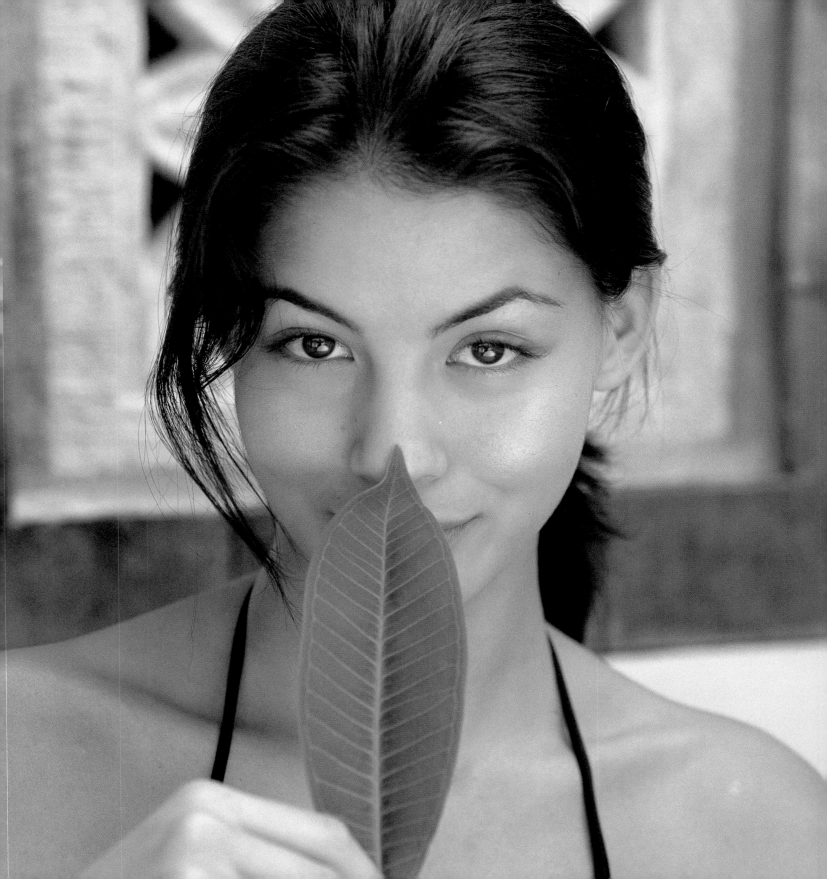

face value

More than any other part of our body, our face reflects most accurately what is going on beneath our skin's façade. It is the clearest indication of the popular maxim: 'beauty from the inside-out'. While we know that we cannot halt our natural ageing process, we can help our skins age with grace by taking a few simple steps. Fresh air, adequate sleep, a high water intake, relaxation and a diet high in fruit and vegetables and low in processed foods, all help our facial skin stay plump and relatively free from blemishes.

Tropical Asian women have a head start on those in the West. These basic steps have been an integral part of their traditional lifestyles for centuries. And many of their facial preparations are mixed directly from the vast botanical heritage that this region lays

claim to. For example, many natural beauty preparations stem from the palaces in Central Java where princesses spent their youth learning and preparing them for their own use. In the absence of night creams, neck creams and new oxygen creams, Asian women have used raw plant extracts to slough off dead skin cells, fight acne, replenish moisture or achieve an SPF.

Now that 'natural' is *de rigueur* once more, women are flocking to Asian spas where traditional treatments, free from clinical input, are giving them soft skin and a relaxed state of mind. 'Back to basics' is the new concept for modern beauty, and ironically, they may now find themselves having their faces 'cleaned' with the very food that, at home, they have hastily wiped from their chins.

Traditional Honey-Cucumber Facial

The principle ingredients of this facial – honey, lime and cucumber – enjoy an age-old reputation as skin healers, softeners and moisturizers. Used in conjunction with each other, these three natural ingredients reduce the discomforts of skin irritations and stem infection while promoting new cell growth.

This simple and sensual facial, offered at *Banyan Tree Spa Bintan* and *Banyan Tree Spa Phuket*, leaves your skin feeling soft and plump and your mind questioning the need for progress in the beauty industry. Who needs electric steamers, electro-magnetic currents, alpha-hydroxy creams for wrinkle reduction and ultimately cosmetic surgery, when nature can be so gentle on the skin and so much kinder on the complexion? Scientific intervention is part of the skincare regimen of the past.

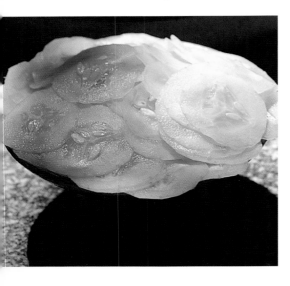

For Scrub

8 oz (1 cup)	clear honey (Thai honey is the most nutritious for this)
10 drops	fresh lime juice
1	medium-sized cucumber, thinly sliced

Steps

1. Cleanse your face with warm water and a natural cloth.
2. Mix the honey and lime juice together and massage into your face for 15 minutes. The sticky-turned-slippery sensation is sublime. The lime peels away surface cells and the honey softens the skin.
3. Wipe away the residue of honey with a wet, warm cloth. Pat dry.
4. Neatly place the cucumber patches over your face and neck (covering eyes and mouth is optional). They feel cool while they tighten the skin and replenish moisture.
5. Finishing with a delicate moisturizer is optional, but not necessary.

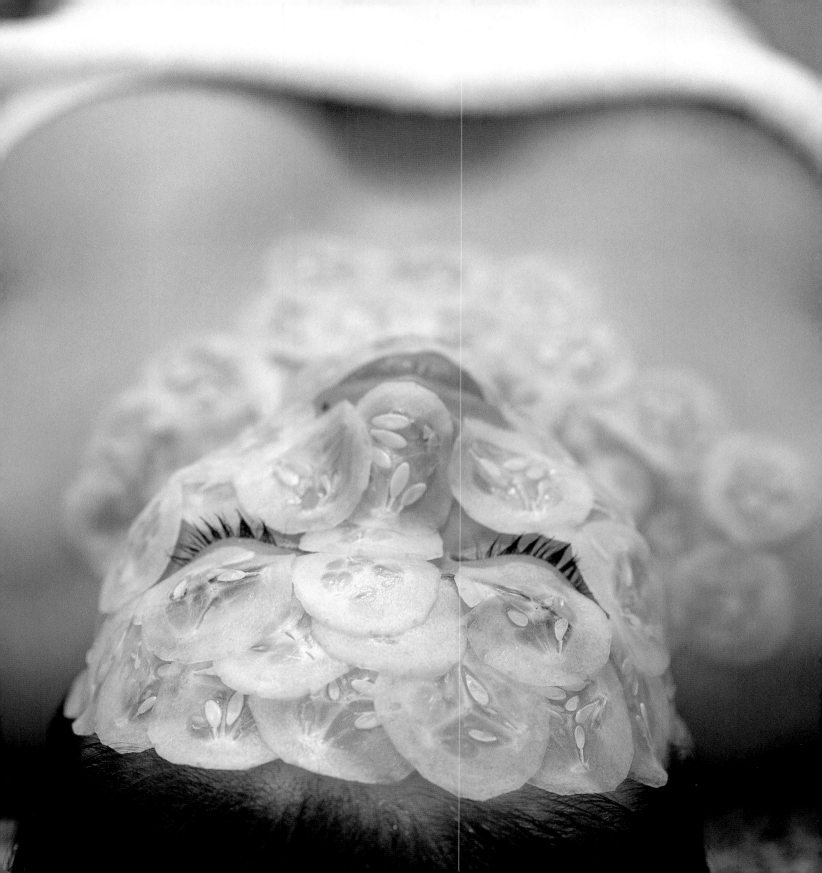

Kitchen Cosmetics

There are all sorts of things in the kitchen cabinets and fridge that can be used for a cleansing and refreshing facial. As part of their five-day Spa Indulgence programme, the *Mandara Spa at The Chedi* in Ubud, Bali, offers an afternoon of practical and fun experiments. Their Kitchen Cosmetics class can be done easily at home as a way of using up what you did not get round to eating. And don't forget that it's only with these sorts of fridge facials that you know *exactly* what you are putting on your skin.

The following can be done in sequence or separately. Word from the 'tried-and-tested' mouths is: "Do these once a month, your skin will feel totally new for three days and will never break out."

Lemon Refresher

Slightly astringent and tightening for the face

1	lemon or lime
¹/₂ tsp	cold water

Mix the lemon or lime juice and the water in a bowl. Gently pat on to your face after any of the treatments on right. The lemon/lime's acidity acts as a toner to tighten the skin and close the pores after a facial. It smells great too!

Egg White Mask

Tightening for a lacklustre complexion

1	egg

Break open the egg and separate the white from the yolk. Beat the white for one minute by hand. Gently apply to the skin and let it harden. Wash off with warm water. The egg white draws toxins from the skin's surface and tightens the pores as it cleans.

Honey Pat

Softening and lifting for the face

2 tbsp	runny honey
2 tsp	lime juice (optional)

Dip your fingers into a bowl containing the honey and lime juice and gently pat onto your skin. Using circular motions, rotate your fingers upward from your chin, cheeks and forehead. Change to a typing motion, tapping the skin and honey until it feels sticky. Let the honey sit for 15 minutes before rinsing off with warm water. Honey is effective in helping your skin to retain moisture.

Polenta and Yoghurt Scrub

Cleansing and exfoliating for face and body

1 tbsp	ground corn meal (polenta)
2 tbsp	natural yoghurt

Mix into a paste and gently rub into your skin, starting at the chin and working up to the cheeks and forehead in small circles. The exfoliating properties of the corn's gritty texture leave your face invigorated and glowing.

Avocado Mask

Softening and nourishing for face and body

1	avocado

Mash the creamy insides into a soft paste and apply to your face using the avocado stone to massage the flesh into your skin with small, upward, circular motions. Wash off with warm water after a few minutes. The nourishing oil is naturally rich in vitamin E and leaves your skin feeling soft.

Traditional Facial

While the concept of the Western facial and its ritual process of toning and scrubbing has no roots in tropical Asian culture, one bumper spa facial combines fresh-from-the-garden produce with some natural skincare products manufactured in Indonesia. This Traditional Facial, found at all Mandara Spas (at *The Chedi*, *Ibah*, *Bali Padma* and *Nikko* in Bali, *Novotel* in Lombok and Malaysia's *The Datai*), includes massage as an unexpected added bonus.

For Scrub

15 gm (1 tbsp)	dry corn kernel
15 gm (1 tbsp)	ground rice powder
15 ml (1 tbsp)	cucumber juice (for oily skin)
or	
15 ml (1 tbsp)	carrot juice (for normal/dry skin)

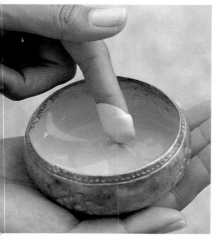

For Mask

20 gm (2 tbsp)	collagen powder (or cosmetic clay powder available at health shops)
10 ml (1 tbsp)	cucumber juice (for oily skin)
or	
10 ml (1 tbsp)	carrot juice (for normal/dry skin)
2	cucumber slices for eyes

For Toning and Moisturizing

Martha Tilaar's *Biokos* cleanser, toner and moisturizer with a seaweed base (*see page 175*)

Steps

1   Mix the corn (dried, yellow kernels) together with the rice powder (finely ground rice). Then add the cucumber or carrot juice to make your scrub.

2   After your cleansing and toning routine (Mandara Spas use the seaweed-rich line *Biokos*, from Martha Tilaar), apply the scrub, taking care not to rub too vigorously as over-zealous rubbing can do more harm than good. Concentrate on the nose area.

3   (While this scrub settles, massage your feet and calves with your favourite oil.)

4   Gently wipe off the scrub, ideally with a natural sponge or muslin cloth dipped in warm water. Tone and moisturize with Martha Tilaar's *Biokos* toner and moisturizer with a seaweed base.

5   Mix the collagen powder (or the cosmetic clay powder, depending on which you use) together with the cucumber or carrot juice to make the mask.

6   Apply the mask with your fingers or a brush and place the cucumber patches over your eyes. (This is where you need a friend who will massage your hands and arms while you drift off under the cooling and tightening mask.)

7   After 15 minutes, gently wipe off the mask with a natural sponge or muslin cloth dipped in warm water.

8   Tone and moisturize and, while massaging the face, skip your fingers over your forehead and cheeks to stimulate your nerve endings.

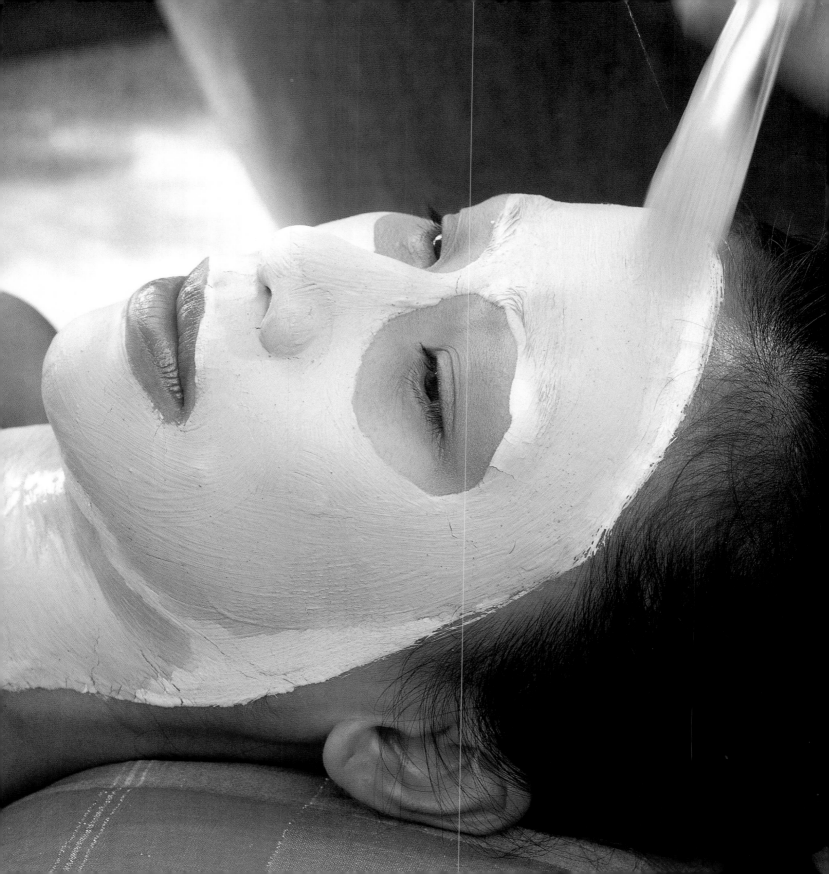

Jamu Tropical Nuts Facial

This facial is fresh from the Indonesian market place and good enough to eat: marzipan scents, cucumber, nuts, lemon grass and warm, melting honey. It was designed especially for *Jamu Body Treatments* in Jakarta according to traditional folklore relating to the medicinal and beautifying agents of local produce. Before doing this facial, prepare the following:

Cucumber Toner

1	small cucumber with skin but not seeds

Blend for 30 seconds. Strain the juice as a toner, but store both the juice and the flesh separately in a fridge.

Almond Milk

20 gms (2 tbsp)	clean, skinned almonds
50 mls (¹/₂ cup)	water

Whiz both in a blender until smooth, about two minutes. Strain several times through a fine mesh cheesecloth to obtain almond milk. Store both the milk and the almond meat in separate containers in the fridge.

City Grime Cleanser

2 tsp	olive oil
1 tsp	thick or runny honey

Mix together.

Kemiri Nut (Candlenut) Milk

For Kemiri Nut Scrub, on right

20 gms (2 tbsp)	*kemiri* nuts
50 mls (¹/₂ cup)	water

Whiz both in a blender until smooth, about two minutes. Strain the mixture several times through a fine mesh cheesecloth until the *kemiri* milk is a silky consistency. Store both the milk and the *kemiri* nut meat in separate containers in the fridge.

Lemon Grass Infusion

For Kemiri Nut Scrub, on right

250 gms (¹/₂ lb)	lemon grass
250 gms (2 cups)	boiling water

Pour the boiling water over the lemon grass. Cover the container and let it stand for 20 minutes until the liquid has cooled down. Strain.

Kemiri Nut (Candlenut) Scrub

10 gms (1 tbsp)	*kemiri* nut meat
1 tsp	*kemiri* nut milk
1 tsp	Lemon Grass Infusion (*see left*)

Mix together into a moist paste. Mix in the Lemon Grass Infusion until the consistency feels right for you.

Almond, Oatmeal and Cucumber Mask

For oily or problem skin

5 cm (2 inches)	unpeeled cucumber
1 tbsp	Almond Milk (*see left*)
40 gms (4 tbsp)	rolled oats
1–2 tbsp	kaolin powder

If you are making this mask separately from the rest of these facial ingredients, blend the cucumber for about 30 seconds, then gently strain the liquid away from the pulp. If you have already made the Cucumber Toner, use the pulp that you have saved from this. Mix all the ingredients together well. Add only enough kaolin powder to make a paste that is dry but workable. The more kaolin used, the faster the mask will dry and the more it will feel tight on your skin.

Avocado, Coconut, Almond and Cucumber Mask

For dry, sun-damaged or ageing skin

5 cm (2 inches)	unpeeled cucumber
1 tbsp	Almond Milk (*see left*)
1/4 fruit	avocado flesh
2 tbsp	coconut oil (or other vegetable oil)
2–3 tbsp	kaolin powder

If you are making this mask separately from the rest of these facial ingredients, blend the cucumber for about 30 seconds, then gently strain the liquid away from the pulp. If you have already made the Cucumber Toner, use the pulp that you have saved from this. Mix all the ingredients together well. Add only enough kaolin powder to make a paste that is dry but workable. The more kaolin used, the faster the mask will dry and the more it will feel tight on your skin.

Steps

1. Clean away any make-up using Cucumber Toner or Almond Milk.
2. Using quick, circular strokes, briskly massage the City Grime Cleanser into the face and neck, concentrating on problem areas.
3. Steam your face and neck with a warm, wet towel and wipe it clean.
4. Apply the Kemiri Nut Scrub to your face using brisk, circular but gentle movements.
5. Wipe off the scrub using a hot, wet towel.
6. Massage your face (and neck and ears) with the Almond Milk. Using your fingers, massage from chin to cheeks to nose to forehead to temples to ears.
7. Steam your face with a hot, wet, towel and wipe away any excess Almond Milk.
8. Cleanse and tone your face with the Cucumber Toner.
9. Apply either the Almond, Oatmeal and Cucumber Mask or the Avocado, Coconut, Almond and Cucumber Mask, depending on your skin type, on both face and neck with a small brush. Leave it for 15–20 minutes.
10. Wipe off the mask using a hot, wet towel and then lay an ice-cold towel on your face. Blot with a tissue.
11. Finish by applying some Cucumber Toner and Almond Milk to re-hydrate the skin.

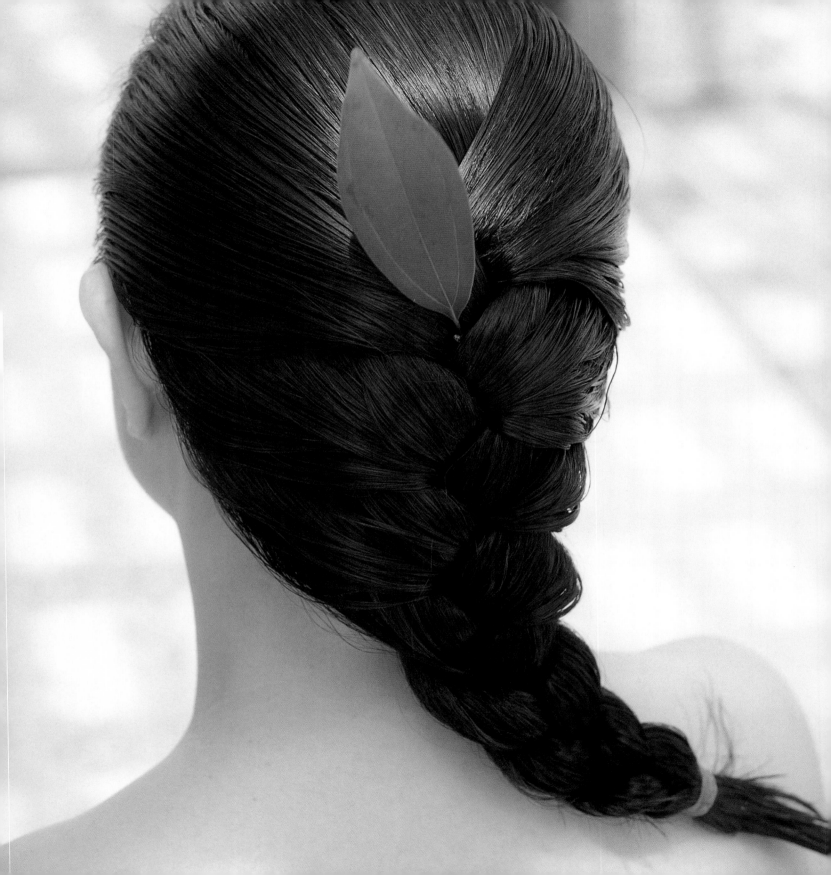

hair story

There is so much truth in the old cliché of 'having a bad hair day'. Feeling bad about the cut, style, touch, bounce and shimmer of our hair – or, more precisely, the lack of these – affects our morale like nothing else. But just like our skin, our hair is a barometer of our general health; it becomes duller and lankier the more tired and poorly nourished we are. It needs fresh air, fresh foods, sleep and low stress levels to maintain its shine. It also depends on a healthy scalp; a good scalp massage activates hair follicles and reduces tension in our heads.

One of the most striking features of tropical Asian women's beauty is their sleek and shiny hair. Historically their locks have been so lustrous precisely because of the lack of detergents available to them and their con-sequent reliance on nature's yield. Today, shampoo has taken over from coconut oil for washing, but hair remains a major focus of beauty ritual, and all manner of natural produce – flowers, oils, plant matter – are regularly applied to keep it glossy. Added to this, the traditional Asian diet based on fruit, vegetables, whole grains and oily fish is perfect nourishment for healthy hair.

While proper cleaning and conditioning provides some of the best protection from environmental attack, manufactured hair products that contain harsh stripping chemicals can do more harm than good. This chapter highlights some more natural remedies, tried and tested by the very women who tout those thick black tresses that speak for themselves.

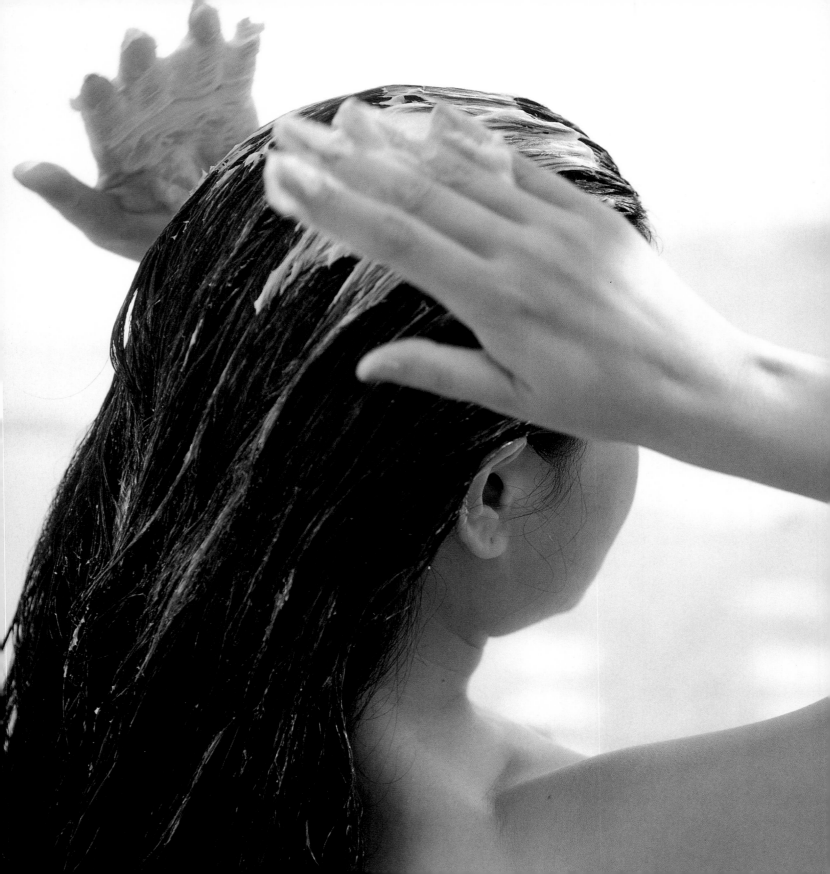

Crème Bath Hair Treatment

The crème bath is synonymous with hair salons everywhere in Asia where hair is a major focus of beauty ritual. It is one of the most popular methods of maintaining the sleek and shiny texture for which Asian women's hair is renowned.

Although often referred to as a 'traditional' head treatment, the crème bath is based on a manufactured product, namely a rich conditioning cream, whose thick glutinous consistency thoroughly coats the hair like icing. After steaming, it is washed off to leave hair superlatively soft and shiny.

Natural ingredients are often added to the crème bath product to treat specific hair conditions. The *St Gregory Javana Spa* in Singapore offers Indonesian-produced hair crèmes for specific hair types for their 90-minute *Mandi Kepala*.

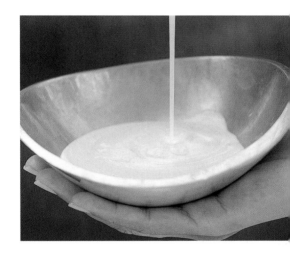

The therapists run their crème-coated fingers through section after section of hair leaving your head feeling cool, clammy, heavy and 'gooey'. Then lie back to the touch of rhythmic finger movements that massage the scalp and gradually move down the neck and shoulders. While you drift off into limbo, the crème is stimulating the scalp and the hair follicles and softening and strengthening the strands of hair.

Natural Crème Bath Additives

Here are some of the flavours recommended for specific hair conditions:

Carrot	for hair growth
Henna	for nourishing dry or permed hair
Avocado	for feeding dry hair
Ginseng	for strengthening the hair roots
Celery	for increasing hair elasticity
Aloe vera	for a general hair food
Candlenut	for promoting glossy, dark hair
Seaweed	for stimulating hair growth
Egg	for healing dry hair and split ends

Aromatherapy Scalp Treatment

This treatment, found exclusively at the *Spa at Bali Hyatt*, Sanur, Bali, must rank among the best head remedies available anywhere. It incorporates a crème bath but also makes use of gels, oils and a heaven-sent massage to awaken your brain, stimulate hair growth and relax the body.

Ingredients

10 mls (1 tbsp)	hot macadamia oil
5 mls (¹/₂ tsp)	essential oil of your choice
3 tbsp	manufactured crème bath

Steps

1. Warm the macadamia oil in an aromatherapy oil burner with your choice of essential oils which are the active ingredients of this treatment (see below). The ratio between base and essential oils should be 2:1. Macadamia oil is used because, unlike the traditional coconut oil, it does not have an aroma that interferes with the scent of the essential oils. The oil is heated so that it penetrates the hair more easily.
2. With your fingers, part the hair. Using a face mask applicator brush, smear the warm oil along the scalp line at one-inch intervals massaging with your finger tips as you go.
3. When your scalp is fairly well covered with oil apply the crème bath from the roots to the ends of your hair and massage your scalp with finger tip pressure. Snap sections of your scalp between fingers and thumb for added stimulation.
4. For best results, cover your head with a loose, clear shower cap and steam for 10–20 minutes, or leave for 20 minutes.
5. Shampoo several times to remove all traces of oil.

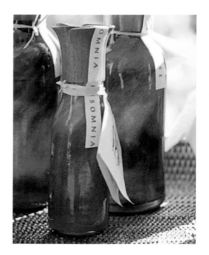

Essential Oils

Best essential oils for the hair as recommended by the *Spa at Bali Hyatt*.

Dry hair	geranium, sandalwood, palmarosa, lavender
Damaged hair	geranium, lavender, sandalwood, frankincense
Blond hair	geranium, lemon, camomile
Grey hair	camomile, sage, lavender, rose
Hair loss	juniper, rosemary, lavender
Dandruff/excema	eucalyptus, rosemary, cedarwood, tea tree

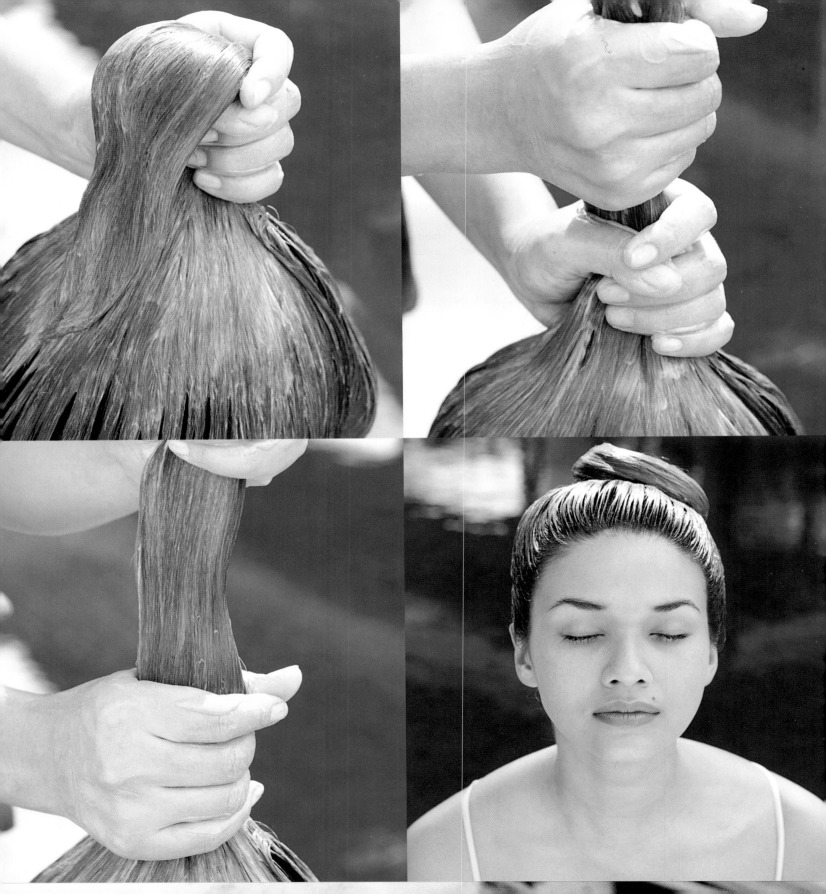

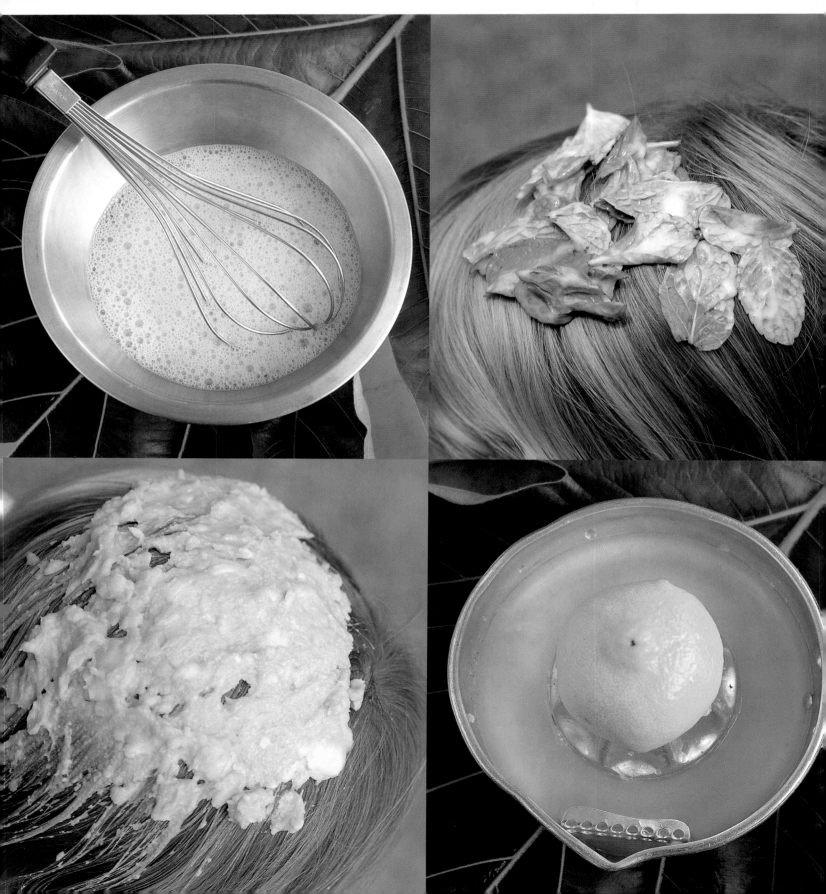

Hair Remedies

For Dry Hair
- Massage the creamy insides of an avocado into clean dry hair and leave for 15–20 minutes.
- Massage coconut oil into your hair and leave for a few hours. Wash several times before your hair feels silky rather than oily.

For Lacklustre Hair
- Massage two large, grated carrots into damp or dry hair. Trap with a bath hat and leave for 15–20 minutes.
- Squeeze half a lemon into 200 mls (1 cup) of water and use the mixture as a final rinse after shampooing.

For Thinning Hair
- Whisk two eggs and massage them into your hair. Wash off after ten minutes to enhance hair growth and strength.
- Put several sticks of celery through a juicer and massage the juice into your scalp. Leave for 15 minutes before washing.

For Dandruff
- Mix a large handful of crushed mint leaves into your conditioner and leave on the hair for 15–20 minutes.

For Fragrant Hair

The sweet-smelling jasmine bud plays an important role in beauty ritual throughout Asia. In Thailand and Indonesia the small flowers are woven into a bride's hair on her wedding day. This type of head-dressing continues among married women in the palaces of Central Java while unmarried women, according to palace tradition, should weave their hair with the fragrant pandanus leaf avoiding any form of flower until she is wed.

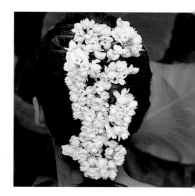

Embrace the exotic and try pinning a few jasmine blooms into your hair as much for the sweet scent as the pretty effect. It is best to plait the hair, thread a classic hairpin through the base of the flower and then wedge the pin into the thick plait of hair.

For Thicker Hair

Aloe vera plants, known in Indonesia as 'alligator's tongue' because of their spiky appearance, grow wild throughout tropical Asia. Their thick spiny leaves contain a cooling sap, which is an elixir for heavy heads. More precisely this extract contains a natural tannin with an anti-inflammatory effect, and saponin, a natural emulsifier.

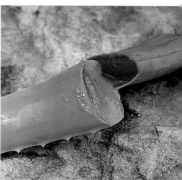

- Break open an aloe vera leaf with a knife to reveal a sticky juice. Massage the juice into the scalp and leave it for 15 minutes. Wash off.
- Feel your scalp cool down and tingle. The aloe's active ingredients stimulate the follicles for a thick and fuller head of hair.

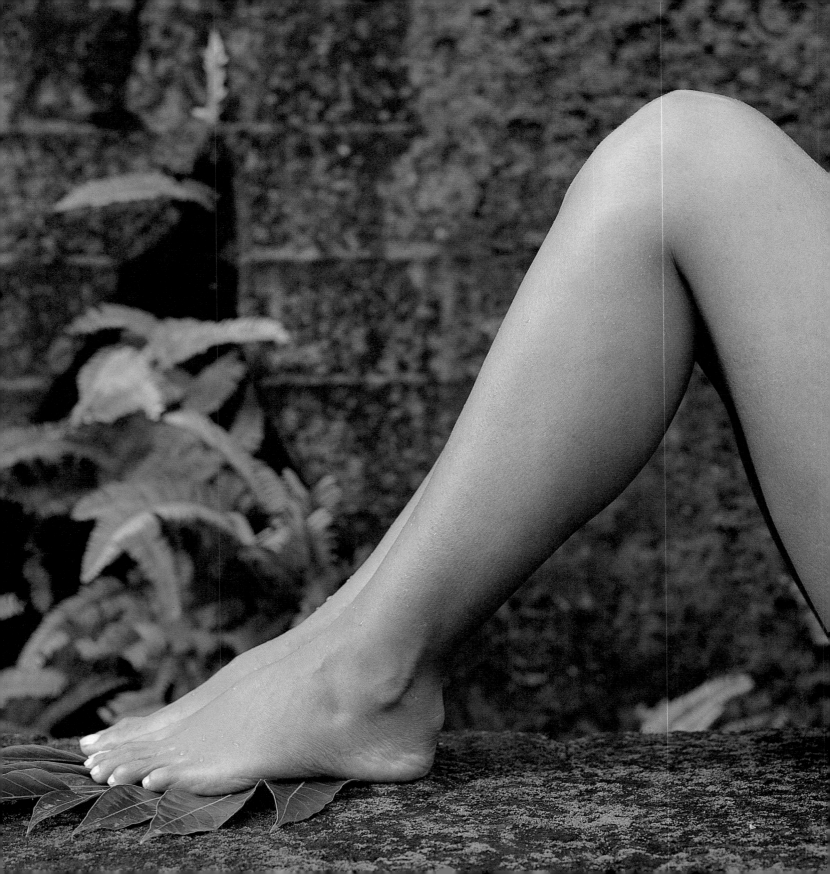

feet first

Of all our body parts, our feet tend to suffer most. They are our trusty servants, yet we stuff them into shoes and pay little respect to the fact that they carry our whole body weight. During our lifetime, they traipse four times around the world or roughly 70,000 miles. In cold weather we ignore them as they are under wraps; when it is hot we pay them scant attention with a swoosh of nail varnish before displaying them in sandals. And we wonder why 'our feet are killing us' as that painful saying goes. There's nothing worse than sore feet, but it is a guaranteed condition if we don't look after them.

Yet our own two feet are crucial in helping us to look after our bodies just by walking. Walking tones our heart and lungs and so boosts our energy. It lowers cholesterol levels, burns calories and therefore helps us to lose weight. Medics also claim that walking reduces the risk of developing osteoporosis, which makes older bones brittle and prone to fracture.

Needless to say, in Asia an ancient technique for foot relief has been practised for centuries. It originated in India and China more than 5,000 years ago and is known loosely as reflexology. It has grown out of the understanding that every part of our faithful pair of feet corresponds to a part of our body, making them key healing zones.

After all, one quarter of all our body's bones (26 different bones) are resident in our feet. It seems they deserve as much, if not more, attention than any other part of our body.

How to...happy feet

Happy feet make happy people. Remember that anointing the feet is a long-held ritual in many cultures. As you rub on these ointments think that you are giving a sacred start – or finish – to your day. This is an almost religious act of gratitude for your mobility! Here are some quick and easy ways to cheer all three of you up.

Pedicure

A pedicure is not simply the pursuit of vanity. A proper one should include a foot soak, a nail trim, which prevents in-growing toenails, and the removal of hard skin and calluses which could, if left, lead to corns. Cuticles should be pushed down, not cut, and feet and calves massaged with cream or oil if skin is particularly dry. An olive oil base is especially nourishing. Painted nails look shiniest and last longest if they get a clear undercoat, two coats of colour and a clear top coat. Polish takes at least 15 minutes to dry.

Most major spas offer a full-on pedicure, although some therapists are more professional than others who can take far too long and poke about in tender spots, so be wary.

Hard Skin

One of the most effective exfoliants for hard skin that develops on the soles of the feet is sand. Collect some ordinary beach sand on your next visit to a tropical spa and mix it with enough vegetable oil to make a sticky paste. Add a few drops of peppermint or rosemary essential oil to complete the invigorating experience. Massage your feet concentrating on the heels, the balls and the big toes where skin is usually hardest.

Quick Tips
1   Cool down hot feet with a peppermint and aloe vera gel rub.
2   Soothe tired feet with a vegetable oil massage spiked with clove oil which has anesthetic properties. Best base oils for feet include avocado, olive and sesame.
3   Soak your feet in warm water laced with pine, tea tree and eucalyptus oils to banish odours.
4   Exercise and strengthen your foot muscles by rolling each foot over a tennis ball while sitting down.
5   Detoxify your whole body with a 10-minute foot soak in warm water containing two tablespoons of rock salt. Follow with an oil massage.
6   Avoid bunions and ankle problems and ditch your high heels. If impossible, wear them sparingly! Keep infections away and change your tights and socks every day. Make sure they, like your shoes, are never too small. Let your feet breathe whenever you can.

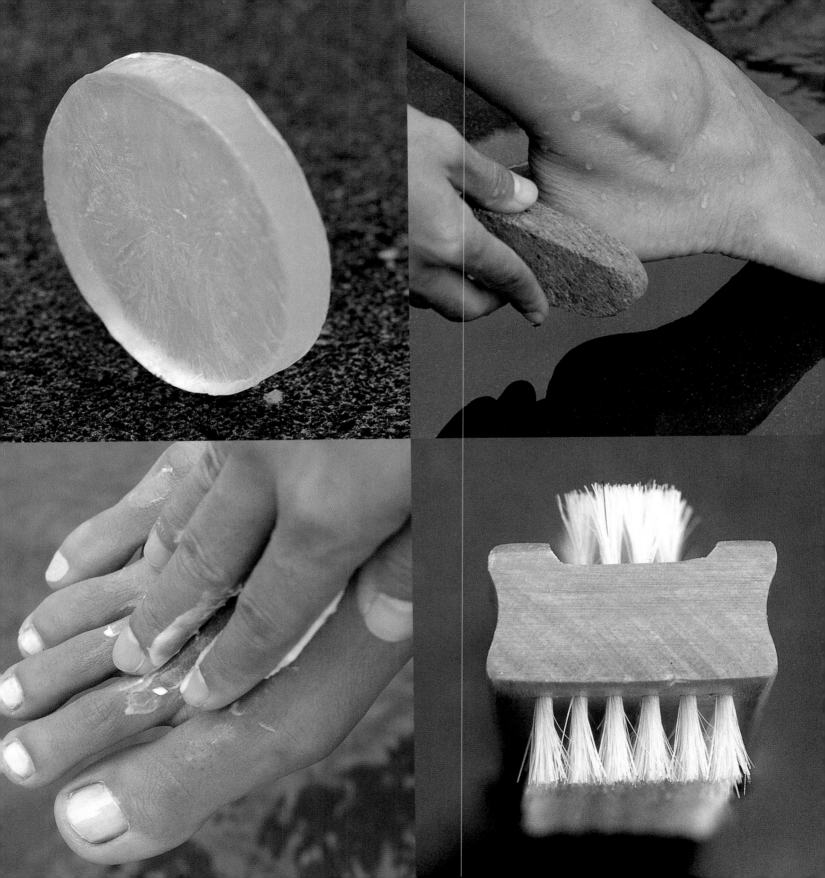

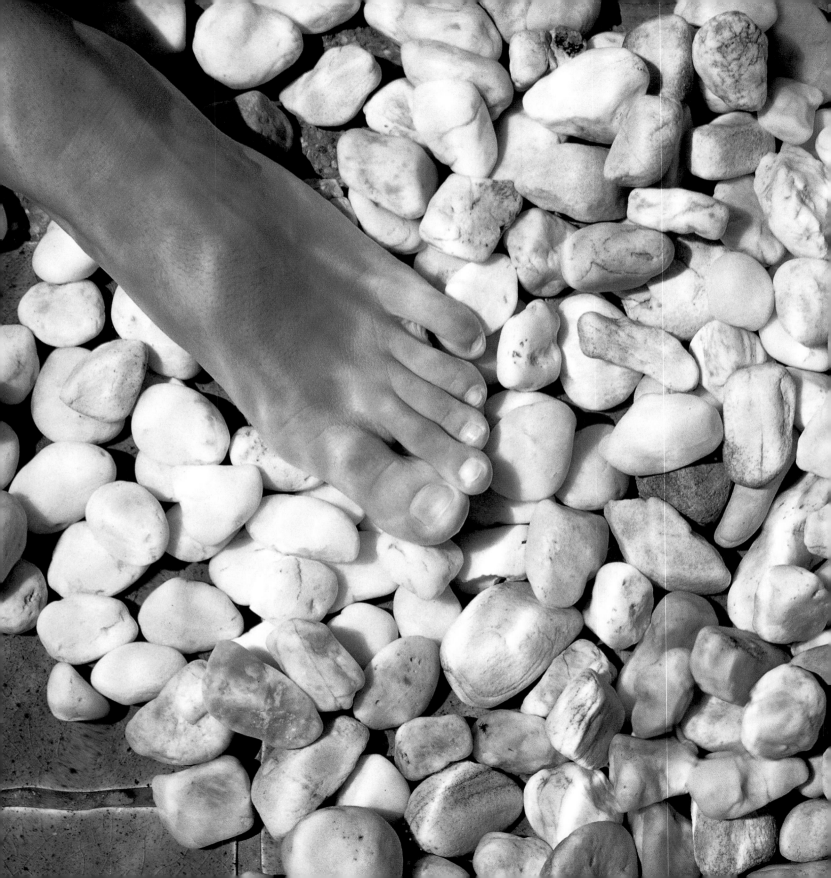

Kneipp Foot Bath

This is a one-off experience on the Asian spa circuit, exclusive to Thailand's *Chiva-Som*. The foot bath itself comprises a corridor, calf-deep with water floating on a bed of stones. The water is cold, the corridor dark and the sensation exhilarating if a little painful on your soles. While it's a relief to step out of the bumpy foot bath onto a flat, dry surface, your feet tingle and your whole body feels alive. You are compelled to walk another circuit, for kicks!

This bath is based on the theory of a 19th-century Bavarian priest, Father Sebastian Kneipp. He systemized the healing properties of water into the science of hydrotherapy and was famous for preaching the health benefits of walking barefoot on dewy morning grass, in keeping with his belief that nature provides us with everything we need to be healthy and happy. At *Chiva-Som*, the foot bath combines the healing powers of water with the principle of reflexology, whereby the sensitive nerve endings in our feet are invigorated by the pressure of the small stones and the cold water.

As a consolation for the wincing you will do, this foot bath encircles *Chiva-Som's* steam bath. Come out of the cold and step into this smoky hot chamber for more body blitzing!

Oriental Foot Massage

Oriental foot massage, otherwise known as reflexology or previously as zone therapy, is an ancient art of healing which works on the principle that the body's organs, including the brain, are connected by energy channels to trigger points in our feet. Consequently, when our feet are tired, so are our minds and bodies.

Reflexologists believe that if a body part (liver, thyroid, gall bladder, eyes and ears) is not functioning properly, the energy flowing through our channels, or meridians, becomes sluggish, even blocked. This can cause crystals to gather under the skin in specific parts of our feet. Massaging these points breaks down the crystals and restores the flow of body energy.

There are reputedly 7,000 nerve endings in our feet and therapists know which area mirrors which body part. Asians are particularly intuitive when it comes to massaging feet and a treatment of this ilk is offered in most spas, either alone or as part of other massage therapies. It is fabulous for stimulating circulation and restoring physical and mental harmony. It is also an uncannily accurate way of both detecting and healing internal problems.

Foot and Nut Treatment

The felons for corns and carbuncles are fashion footwear, tights and high heels, all of which we thrust upon our faithful feet. Give them time out and treat them to a weekly foot soak and massage, but if you find yourself in Bali, do not leave until your trotters have tried this bumper foot treatment at *Jamu Traditional Spa*, Kuta. They never knew life could be so good. If you are doing this Foot and Nut Treatment at home, prepare the following before starting:

Honey Milk Cleansing Lotion

10 pieces	*kemiri* nut (candlenut)
3 tbsp	honey
4 tbsp	water

Blend the *kemiri* nuts and water together for two minutes. Using a fine mesh cheesecloth strain the milk from the meat. Save the meat for the Kemiri Nut Scrub and two tablespoons of the milk for the flower mask. Add the honey to the milk and mix well. This is now ready to use.

Lemon Grass Infusion

For Kemiri Nut Scrub, on right

250 gms (¹/₂ lb)	lemon grass
250 gms (2 cups)	boiling water

Pour the boiling water over the lemon grass. Cover the container and let it stand for 20 minutes until the liquid has cooled down. Strain.

Kemiri Nut Scrub

as saved	*kemiri* nut meat
500 gms (2 cups)	Lemon Grass Infusion

Use the nut meat already prepared for the cleansing lotion and mix it with enough of the Lemon Grass Infusion to make a moist paste that can be sensually rubbed into your feet.

Flower Mask

5 tbsp	kaolin powder
2 tbsp	*kemiri* nut milk
1 tsp	ground cinnamon
1 tsp	ground cloves
1 tsp	ground ginger
handful	pandanus leaves, hibiscus, frangipani or other delicate flowers such as rose, finely chopped
5 drops	lavender essential oil

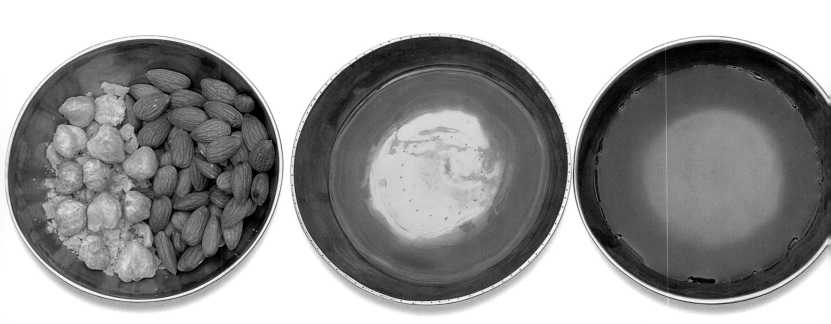

Mix kaolin powder, *kemiri* nut milk, ground cinnamon, cloves and ginger, pandanus leaves or flower, and lavender essential oil together into a paste that is dry but workable. The more kaolin used the faster the mask will dry and the cooler it will feel on your feet.

Steps

1   Wash your feet in a tub with a few drops of your favourite essential oil. Make sure you dry them properly between the toes and outwards along the nail growth on the side of each toe, removing all moisture so as to avoid infection.

2   Using cotton wool, rub the Honey Milk Cleansing Lotion all over each foot. The nut content is both astringent and deeply moisturizing while the honey both exfoliates some of the finer dead skin and softens it.

3   Relish rubbing your feet with the Kemiri Nut Scrub trapping the grains between your thumb and the nerve endings in the soles of your feet – there are over 7,000 of them! This very sensuous step leaves your feet wide awake and tingling.

4   Wipe away the scrub with a warm cloth and remove the finer traces with some more Honey Milk Cleansing Lotion.

5   Scoop the Flower Mask into the palm of your hands and pat it around your feet, covering them entirely up to the ankle to make two clay booties. It is best to sit back with your feet up on a stool covered with a towel. Enjoy the tightening and cooling sensation. Leave for 20 minutes before washing off with warm water.

6   Finish off with a calming aromatic foot massage using a rich carrier oil such as avocado, sesame or olive, plus a few drops of your favourite essential oil.

This is quite a labour-intensive treatment if done at home, but leaves your feet feeling loose and fluid. It is altogether a more divine experience at *Jamu Traditional Spa* where you sit back under the dappled shade of a banyan tree. Here therapists treat your calves as well as your feet. Both are cosseted for an hour and a half.

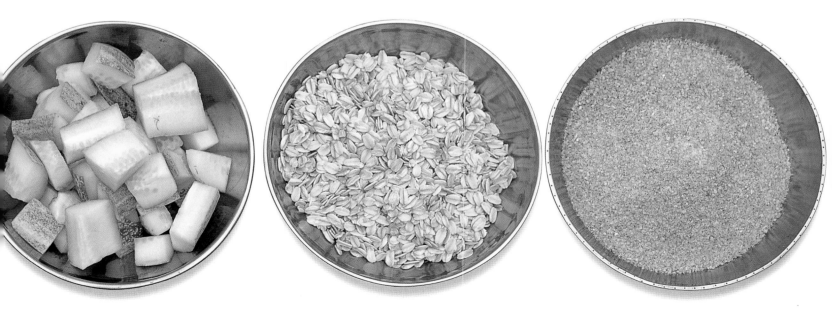

Floral Foot Soak

Soaking feet in warm water is an ancient form of pain relief practised, in varying guises, throughout many cultures. For centuries people have dissolved Epsom salts to reduce swelling, rock salt to detoxify the whole body at bedtime, or peppermint oil to cool and tickle the nerve endings.

In Bali, the higher castes allegedly keep a bowl of water in the corner of their bedroom, filled with flowers and the oil of eucalyptus for a ritual cleansing at the end of the day. Foot washing is also a symbolic part of one of the many rites of passage in Balinese Hinduism, carried out as a sign of deference to Sang Hyang Widhi, one of the gods responsible for the order of balance and imbalance in our lives.

You can experience the most heavenly foot soak in Bali at the *Spa at Bali Hyatt* where it is given as a matter of course before every treatment. You don't even have to lift your foot in or out of the thick wooden tub!

The treatment consists of gentle splashing with the scented flower water and gentle skin sloughing with volcanic stone: soft, white stone for women and a coarser black one for men. After this, heavy feet shed tension and start floating. After patting them dry, your therapist will massage your feet and legs with oil, working up toward the heart, using her thumb and forefinger to apply pressure up the back of the calf from the ankle. According to massage theory these strokes relieve poor circulation, fluid retention and bladder problems. The whole experience is so pleasurable and focused (and it could never last long enough!) that it hardly matters what, if any, medical benefits are taking place.

Use essential oils in your own foot soak. The *Spa at Bali Hyatt* favours three drops each of thyme, vetiver and sage as a good combination to make skin smooth. Flowers are added as a symbolic gesture to wash away bad luck. As an intrinsic part of every day life in Asia, flowers represent a bridge to the natural world, taking on a spiritual and cleansing significance. Don't make the water too hot and soak for 10–15 minutes for best results. Follow by massaging your feet with a rich oil such as coconut, olive or avocado.

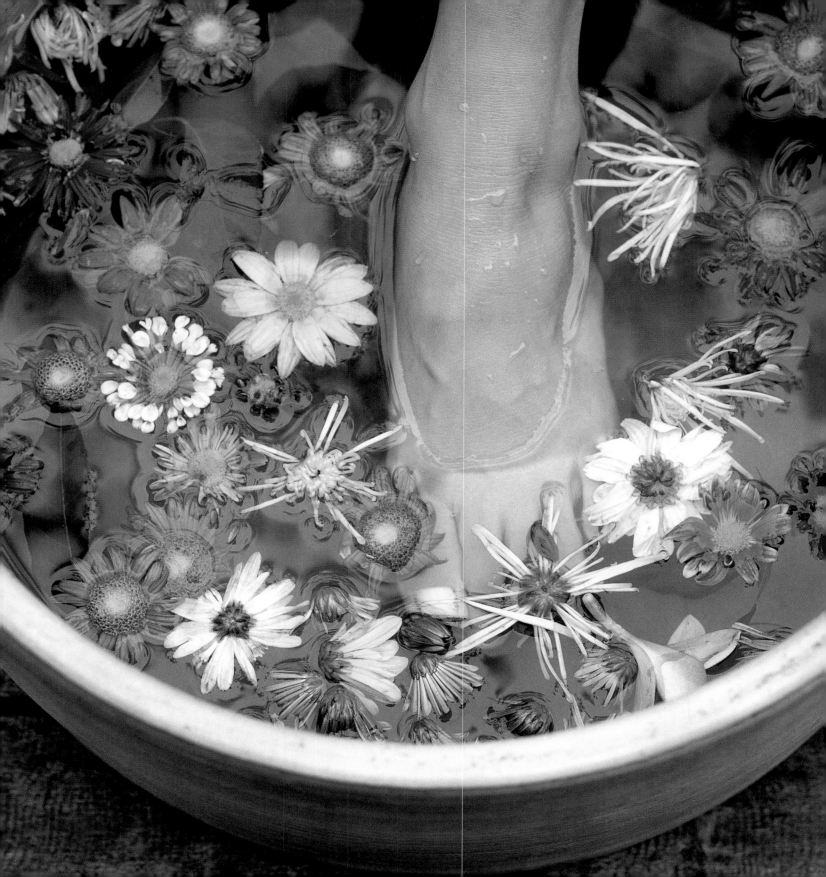

asian spa
cuisine

We have all heard the maxim 'we are what we eat'. Southeast Asian spa cuisine adds a bit of oriental pizzazz to healthy dining choices.

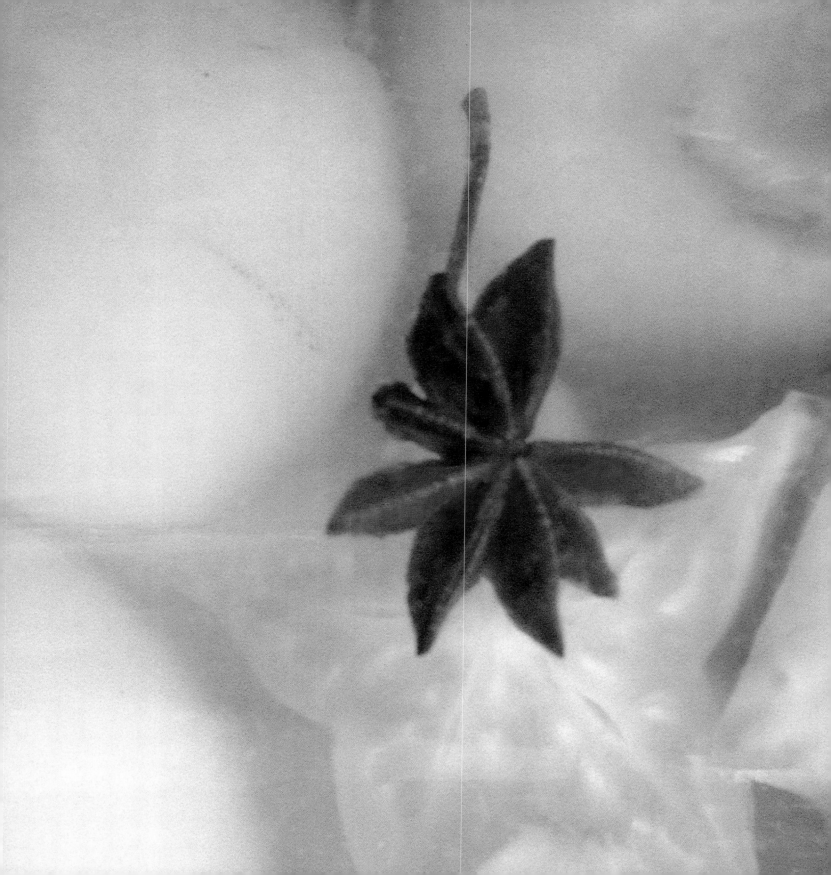

A Kickstart to the Day

As the years roll by, people the world over are getting fatter. This is not because we are eating more. Surveys show that generally people are eating less; they are just eating badly. One of the prime culprits of this is skipping breakfast in the mad dash for the office; culprit number two: a sedentary lifestyle.

When we skip meals we send our bodies into starvation mode forcing them to store up the energy they are not getting and making us feel lethargic as a result. Instead we should eat little and often and prepare our bodies for the rigours of the day with a sensible breakfast that contains unrefined starches, for example the whole grains in muesli. These may take some time for the body to digest, but the nutrients in them are easily absorbed releasing steady levels of energy throughout the day. What's more, people who eat lots of starchy, fibrous foods, including fruit and vegetables, have a lower risk of both heart disease and cancer. Here are some healthy breakfast options, from the *Nusa Dua Spa* in Bali.

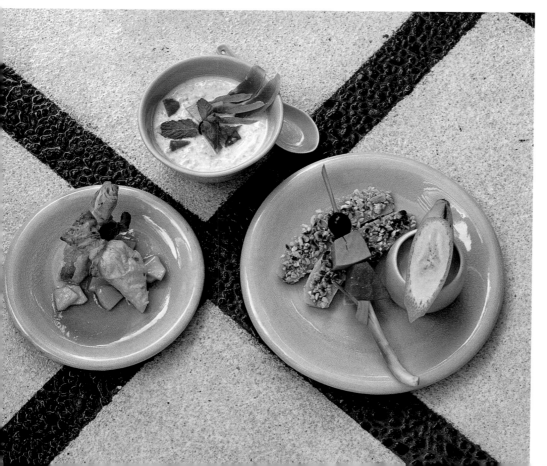

Asian Golden Muesli
(serves four)

250 gms (1 cup)	Swiss muesli
600 ml (3 cups)	soy milk
100 gms (¹/₂ cup)	plain yoghurt
150 gms (³/₄ cup)	papaya, chopped
150 gms (³/₄ cup)	mango, chopped
100 gms (¹/₂ cup)	fructose
juice of 4	limes, juiced
100 gms (¹/₂ cup)	honey
2 ml (1 tsp)	pandan essence (*krim bai toey*, sold at Thai grocery stores)

Method Mix all the ingredients together, then pour into a medium-sized bowl. The mixture can be stored for four hours before serving. If the mixture is a little dry, add more soy milk, then garnish with dry sweet papaya and dry mango and mint leaves.

Grilled Banana with Cashew Nuts and Honey served with Fresh Fruit
(serves four)

4	bananas
80 gms (¹/₄ cup)	honey
88 gms (¹/₄ cup)	cashew nuts, chopped
120 gms (¹/₂ cup)	plain yoghurt
4 gms (2 tsp)	dextrose
40 gms (¹/₄ cup)	tangerine juice
4 sticks	lemon grass
80 gms (¹/₂ cup)	papaya, chopped
60 gms (¹/₂ cup)	watermelon, chopped
20 gms (¹/₄ cup)	grapefruit sections

Method Slice the bananas in half and grill until they are a little soft. Brush with honey and sprinkle with chopped cashew nuts. Grill again until golden brown. Place on a dessert plate with plain yoghurt and the tangerine juice and dextrose mix. Skewer the fresh fruit on to the lemon grass stick, place on the side and serve immediately.

Apple Strudel with Honey
(serves four)

175 gms (2 cups)	apple, chopped
50 gms (6 tbsp)	fructose
2 gms (1 tsp)	cinnamon
40 gms (¹/₄ cup)	raisins
3 gms (2 tsp)	lime juice
2 gms (1 tsp)	zest of lime
25 gms (2 tbsp)	honey
100 gms (1 cup)	breadcrumbs
40 gms (¹/₂ cup)	almonds, ground
25 gms (2 tbsp)	butter
dash	vanilla essence
180 gms (¹/₄ lb)	filo pastry dough
1	egg, lightly whisked

For the Apple Sauce

50 gms (¹/₄ cup)	apple juice
40 gms (¹/₄ cup)	fructose
25 gms (2 tbsp)	honey
5 gms (1 tsp)	flour
50 gms (³/₄ cup)	apple, chopped
60 gms (6 tbsp)	water

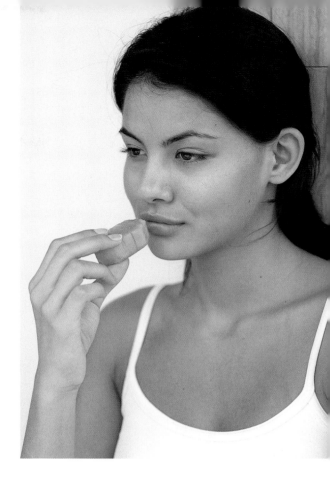

Method Mix all the ingredients, with the exception of the pastry and the egg. Unroll the filo pastry which should be four layers thick. Cut the pastry into four squares. Divide the filling into four parts. Place a ¹/₄ of the filling in the centre of each pastry square. Brush with the egg, then bake for 20 minutes in a preheated oven at 325°F (160°C).

For the sauce, mix all the ingredients together in a food processor. Serve with the apple strudel when fully baked.

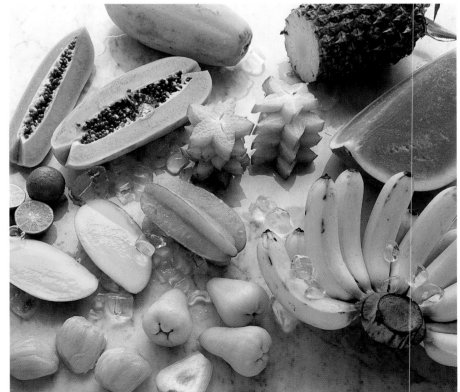

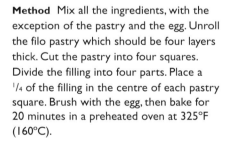

Simple Food

After your body has gone through the rigours of massage it is advisable to eat simple food that is easily digestible. Your digestive system is also much more responsive when you are feeling calm. At *The Serai* in east Bali, the chef creates tasty recipes that require little cooking. These dishes are healthy post-massage snacks that are light without being insubstantial.

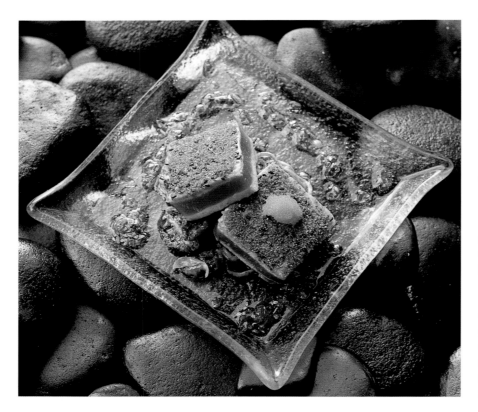

Tuna with Coriander and Ginger Dressing, and Spinach Noodles
(one serving)

1 (6–8 oz)	tuna steak
1 recipe	Pepper Mix (see below)
1 tbsp	vegetable oil
90 gms (¼ lb)	spinach noodles
1 recipe	Coriander and Ginger Dressing (see below)
small bunch	chopped coriander

Pepper Mix Mix together the following: 1 tbsp Cajun spice, 1 tbsp whole black sesame seeds, 1 tbsp (less if dried) fresh oregano, 1 tsp garlic powder, 1 tbsp (less if dried) roasted ground coriander seeds, 1 tsp roasted ground fennel seeds.

Coriander and Ginger Dressing Mix together the following: 4 slices ginger, 450 mls (¾ cup) olive oil, 30 mls (1 tbsp) rice wine vinegar, 30 mls (1 tbsp) Mirin (rice wine), 1 clove garlic, salt and pepper to taste.

Method Coat the tuna steak in the Pepper Mix and pan fry in hot vegetable oil for approximately two minutes each side. Blanch the noodles, for about two minutes in boiling water. Drain them well. Serve the tuna on top of the noodles and coat with the Coriander and Ginger Dressing and chopped coriander.

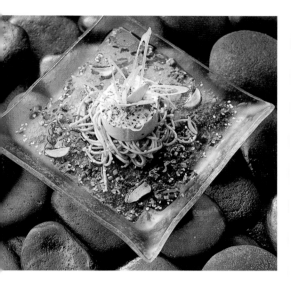

Silken Tofu

(one serving)

75 gms (¹/₂ cup)	blanched buckwheat soba noodles
1 recipe	Japanese Ponzu Sauce
half	small red chilli, sliced
1 tsp	sesame oil
1 tsp	lime juice
3 slices	silken tofu (about ¹/₂ cup)
half	leek, sliced, fried in vegetable oil until crispy
pinch	ground black pepper
small bunch	chopped coriander

Ponzu Sauce Ponzu is a Japanese citrus sauce available in Asian-style grocery stores. Mix one part Ponzu with one part Mirin (rice wine) and one part soy sauce, some crispy fried garlic (do it with the leeks), 1 tbsp olive oil and salt and pepper to taste.

Method Soak the noodles in half of the Ponzu sauce, then add the sesame oil and lime juice and half the chopped coriander. Place the sliced silken tofu on top of the noodles and garnish with the crispy leeks, ground black pepper, rest of the chopped coriander and the remaining Ponzu sauce.

Rucola (Rocket or Arugula) Salad

(one serving)

¹/₂ cup	Parmesan cheese, grated
handful	fresh rucola leaves
1 recipe	Balsamic Dressing (see below)

Balsamic Dressing Mix together 150 mls (6 tbsp) olive oil, 50 mls (2 tbsp) balsamic vinegar, ¹/₂ tsp puréed fresh garlic, salt and pepper to taste.

Method Arrange the grated Parmesan cheese in a rectangle shape roughly 8 cm by 4 cm (4 inches by 2 inches) on grease-proof paper. Bake in a preheated 350°F (170°C) oven until the cheese is golden brown, about 10 minutes. While the cheese is still hot, wrap it around a wine bottle or soft drinks can so it dries in a cylindrical shape; remove when it is cool and firm. Arrange the rucola leaves in the cheese basket; drizzle with the Balsamic Dressing.

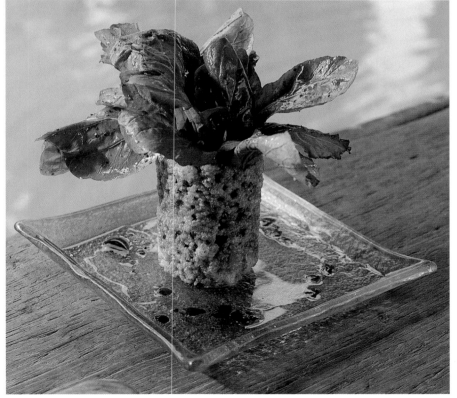

A Natural Feast

One of the many delights of tropical Asia is dining *al fresco*. Food somehow tastes better eaten under a grass roof open at the sides to make the most of a warm evening breeze. At *Begawan Giri Estate* in Ubud, outdoor dining is taken one step further. Order a designer picnic and find a secluded spot amongst some of Bali's most dramatic, landscaped scenery.

Here, a poolside snack is given new meaning. Chips and pizza wedges round the lap pool are swapped for a bit of banana blossom and a bamboo salad at the edge of a jungle rock pool, fed via a waterfall from a 'holy' spring. You feel like a wood nymph as you nibble away in nirvana!

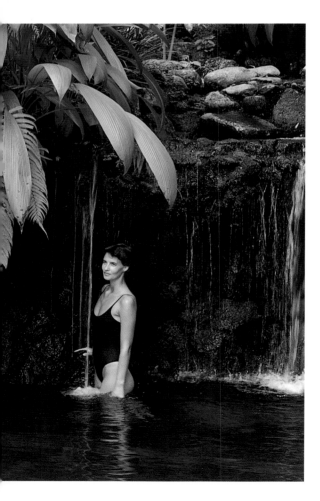

Asparagus and Oyster Mushroom Salad

(one serving)

4 spears	asparagus
6	oyster mushrooms
60 gms (4 tbsp)	fresh coconut, shredded
60 gms (4 tbsp)	lemon grass, finely sliced
15 gms (1 tbsp)	lime leaves, finely sliced
15 gms (1 tbsp)	red shallots, finely sliced
60 gms (4 tbsp)	mint leaves
60 gms (4 tbsp)	coriander leaves
1 recipe	Dressing (see below)
2 gms (½ tbsp)	sesame seeds
2	starfruit leaves (or basil leaves), crisply fried

Dressing

60 gms (4 tbsp)	coconut cream
30 gms (2 tbsp)	Chilli Jam (see right)
15 gms (1 tbsp)	palm sugar
30 gms (2 tbsp)	fish sauce (*nam pla*)
2 small	green chillies, sliced
2 tbsp	Kaffir lime or kalamansi lime juice

To make the Dressing Lightly whisk all ingredients together.

To make Chilli Jam Fry, in 60 ml (4 tbsp) grapeseed oil, 60 gms (4 tbsp) sliced red shallots, and strain; then 30 gms (2 tbsp) sliced garlic; then 15 gms (1 tbsp) dried shrimps; 15 gms (1 tbsp) de-seeded dried chilli (for only 10 seconds). Slice 5 gms (1 tbsp) galangal (or ginger, as a substitute) and pan-toast until perfumed and slightly charred. Cool these ingredients, then blend or purée together with the strained oil. Return the paste to a pot and cook until aromatic and a deep shiny black colour.

Finally, season with 20 gms (1½ tbsp) fish sauce (*nam pla*), 15 ml (1 tbsp) palm sugar and 15 ml (1 tbsp) tamarind water (this is obtained by covering tamarind pulp with warm/hot water, allowing it to seep for 30 minutes, then literally pushing the solids through a strainer). A jam consistency will now have been achieved.

Method Blanch asparagus in chicken stock or water and slice into three pieces. Char-grill the oyster mushroom. To assemble, tumble all the ingredients together, add the Dressing and sprinkle with sesame seeds and crisply fried starfruit leaves.

Crisp Banana Blossom and Green Apple Salad

(one serving)

60 gms (4 tbsp)	banana blossom
60 gms (4 tbsp)	green apple, julienned
15 gms (1 tbsp)	red shallot, sliced
15 gms (1 tbsp)	red shallot, char-grilled
15 gms (1 tbsp)	mint leaves
15 gms (1 tbsp)	coriander leaves
15 gms (1 tbsp)	sliced garlic, crisp-fried
15 gms (1 tbsp)	sliced shallot, crisp-fried
1 recipe	Batter (see below)
1 recipe	Dressing (see below)

Batter Mix together 12 gms (8 tbsp) rice flour, 60 gms (4 tbsp) corn flour, 120 ml (8 tbsp) water and a pinch of salt.

Dressing

1	large red chilli
60 gms (4 tbsp)	lime juice
60 gms (4 tbsp)	orange juice
15 gms (1 tbsp)	white sugar
15 ml (1 tbsp)	fish sauce (*nam pla*)

To make the Dressing Pound in a mortar and pestle the large red chilli until fine. Add all remaining ingredients, stand for 10 mins, stirring lightly on occasion.

Method Top off the round end of the banana flower and peel down the red outer leaves until the white heart appears. Slice it lengthways into four and remove from each piece the hard inner stem. Shake out the flower spores between each layer. Slice the blossom very finely lengthways, working quickly to avoid discolouration. Immediately place in the batter and fry in hot oil over a high heat. Lift out and drain. Finish the salad, by folding all ingredients together.

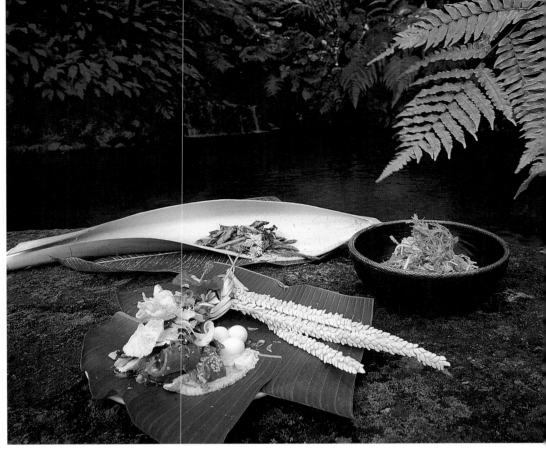

Bamboo, Eggplant and Quail Eggs with a Peanut Relish

(one serving)

1	capsicum
1	baby eggplant
3	quail eggs
30 gms (2 tbsp)	fresh bamboo, cooked in water for 30-40 mins
20 gms (1½ tbsp)	silken tofu, uncooked
1 tsp	fried crisp shallots
60 gms (4 tbsp)	snake beans, blanched in salted water
4	melinjo nut wafers
1 recipe	Peanut Relish

Peanut Relish Blend together 400 gms (2 cups) char-grilled red shallots, 400 gms (2 cups) char-grilled garlic, 60 gms (¼ cup) finely chopped galangal, 120 gms (½ cup) finely chopped lemon grass, 1 large dried chilli soaked in hot water for 30 mins, and then fry with a little vegetable oil for 40 minutes on a low heat. Add 1 cup peanuts, boiled for 10 mins and strained, 1 tsp lime juice and 1 tsp dark palm sugar.

Method Peel and de-seed the capsicum and char-grill. Slice and deep-fry the eggplant. Soft boil the eggs for 2½ minutes. Place the peanut relish on the plate then layer with the above ingredients, followed by the bamboo, tofu, shallots and beans, adding the melinjo wafers at the end.

Tasteful Thai

Guests at *Chiva-Som* have no choice but to reassess their eating habits. Everyone here is presented with a low-fat, no-salt menu three times a day. While Thai food has historically been healthy, it has developed over the years to rely heavily on fat-filled coconut milk, coconut oil and pork meat. *Chiva-Som*'s healthy alternatives are high on flavour and low on these villains. Salt is substituted with soy or fish sauce (*nam pla*) and frying is done with vegetable stock rather than with oil. When using vegetable stock continue adding two tablespoons throughout the cooking process, maintaining the same high heat as if using oil. Here's how:

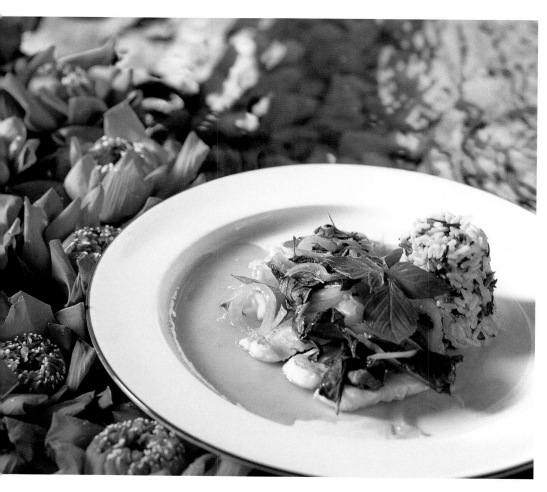

Stir Fried King Fish Thai Style
(serves four)

600 gms (1½ lb)	king fish fillet (or other white fish)
2 cloves	garlic
1	small onion
2	green chilli or red chilli
2 tsp	fresh Thai basil
150 mls (½ cup)	vegetable stock
2 tbsp	fish sauce (*nam pla*) or light soy sauce
200 gms (1 cup)	brown rice

Method Steam the brown rice until crispy, but not overcooked. Cut the fish into medallions, about 1 cm x 3 cm. Crush the garlic and peel and shred the onion. Finely slice the green chilli (or shred the red chilli depending on what you use). Heat a wok or heavy frying pan until hot (but not smoking). Add 50 ml of the stock, the shredded onion and crushed garlic and cook quickly, stirring continuously to prevent burning. If this becomes too dry add a little more stock. Add the fish and continue to stir for 3–4 minutes, taking care not to break up the fish. Continue to add a little stock if the mixture becomes too dry. Add the chilli and basil with the fish sauce. Mix well to coat the fish and serve with the brown rice.

Thai Seafood Salad

(serves four)

4 cloves	garlic
12	bird's-eye chillis
8 tbsp (¹/₄ cup)	lemon juice
4 tsp	fish sauce (*nam pla*)
I tsp	honey
4 thin strips	lemon grass
400 gms (I lb)	mixed, cooked seafood
4	tomatoes
2 stalks	celery
I	large onion
4	spring onions
40 gms (2 tbsp)	Chinese parsley (cilantro)

Method Crush the garlic and chilli together. Add the fish sauce, lemon juice, sliced lemon grass and honey. Set aside. Mix the cooked seafood with the finely shredded celery and onion, seeded and sliced tomato, spring onions and parsley, then mix together with the dressing. Serve immediately.

Lentil Wontons with Sweet and Sour Sauce, Thai Style

(serves four)

75 gms (I cup)	dry lentils
2 tsp	soy sauce
3	spring onions, chopped
¹/₂ tsp	fresh, grated ginger
32	wonton wrappers
I recipe	Sweet and Sour Sauce
750 ml (2¹/₂ cups)	vegetable stock

Sweet and Sour Sauce

125 mls (¹/₂ cup)	vegetable stock
¹/₄	pineapple, diced
¹/₄	cucumber, seeded and diced
¹/₂	bell pepper, chopped
2	tomatoes, seeded
I	spring onion, chopped
2	small chilli
2 tsp	soy sauce
¹/₂ tsp	corn starch
to taste	salt and pepper

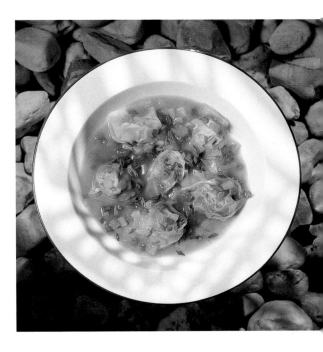

Method Cook the lentils, then mash the cooked lentils in a bowl and add the soy, spring onions and ginger. Place a tea-spoonful in the centre of each wonton wrapper and fold up, moistening the edges with water to seal and shape. Blanch these for 2–3 minutes. Meanwhile, mix the sauce ingredients. Boil the wontons in the vegetable stock, cooking thoroughly for 2–3 minutes. Drain and place in the centre of a plate. Pour over the sauce to serve.

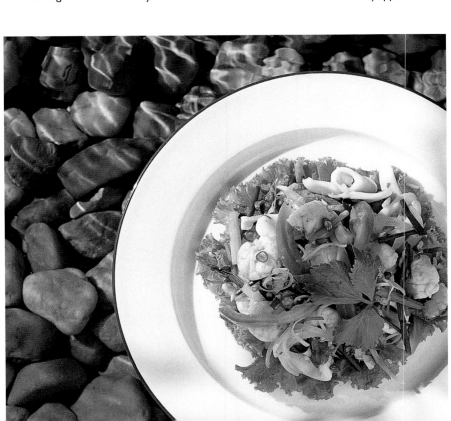

Dining Light

Not many of us manage to stick by the rules of healthy eating, especially when it comes to dinner which, nutritionists tell us, should be eaten at least three hours before bedtime. However we can avoid system overload in our slumbering hours by eating sensibly after dark. This means eating foods that are easily digestible, foods that are as near to their natural state as possible and foods that, if not raw, are lightly cooked: preferably steamed or grilled so that their nutrients are not zapped or strangled by heavy sauces. We should put a hold on our portion size, eat slowly and masticate!

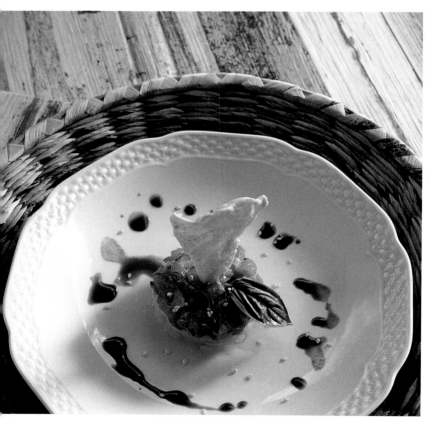

Don't worry about clock watching if you take this evening meal on the lip of Ayung River Gorge at The Chedi in Ubud, Bali, where the location alone will set you up to eat properly – and slowly – and sleep blissfully afterwards.

Tuna Tartar With Cucumber Yoghurt Sauce
(one serving)

75 gms (3 oz)	fresh red tuna (sashimi grade)
20 gms (1 tbsp)	pickled ginger slices
1 tsp	fresh ginger juice, squeezed from grated ginger
3–4 (¼ cup)	spring onions, chopped into small rings
⅛ tsp	Wasabi paste
1 tbsp	soy sauce
1 recipe	Cucumber Yoghurt Sauce (see below)
to garnish	shredded cucumber, sesame seed cracker, sesame seeds

Cucumber Yoghurt Sauce Mix together 1 tbsp yoghurt, 2 tbsp puréed cucumber (seeds removed), salt and pepper to taste.

Method Cut the tuna into small cubes. Mix the Wasabi paste and soy sauce until smooth. Toss the tuna with the Wasabi and soy and the other ingredients until well mixed. On a plate pack the shredded cucumber garnish half way up a metal or pastry ring. Tightly stack the tuna mixture on top to form a cylindrical structure. Pour a circle of cucumber yoghurt sauce around the tuna. Remove the ring. Sprinkle with sesame seeds and serve with a sesame seed cracker on top.

Grilled Chicken Teriyaki and Spicy Noodle Salad

(one serving)

150 gms (5 oz)	chicken breast, boneless and skinless
125 gms ($^1/_2$ cup)	soba noodles
30 gms (2 tbsp)	carrots, shredded
25 gms ($^1/_4$ cup)	broccoli florets
15 gms ($^1/_2$)	leek, julienned
20 gms (2 tbsp)	snowpea pods
15 gms (1 tbsp)	pickled ginger, julienned
$^1/_8$ tsp	Wasabi paste
5 gms (2 tbsp)	nori, shredded in strips
1 recipe	Teriyaki Sauce (see below)
1 recipe	Dressing (see below)

Teriyaki Sauce Mix together 7 tsp soy sauce, 2 tsp sugar, 1 tsp chopped garlic, 1 tsp chopped ginger, 7 tsp Saké and 7 tsp Mirin.

Dressing Mix together 1 tbsp rice vinegar, 1 tbsp Kikkoman soy sauce, 2 tbsp Mirin, 1 tbsp sesame oil, 1 tsp Saké and 2 tbsp chilli oil.

Method Marinate the chicken breast in the Teriyaki Sauce for at least two hours. Cook the noodles until al dente, approximately two minutes. Cool them down in iced water and drain them. Keep aside. Blanch all the vegetables. Grill the chicken breast and slice. Toss the noodles with the vegetables, pickled ginger and Wasabi. Pile them all into a spiral. Top with the chicken pieces and nori strips and sprinkle Dressing and sesame seeds on top.

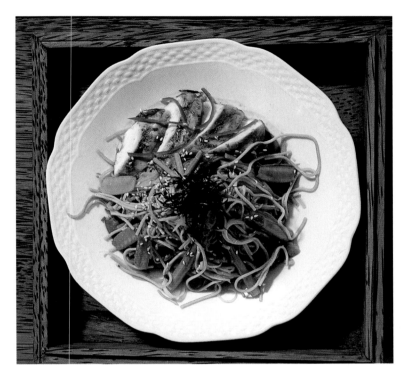

Grilled Fruit Skewers with Honey Yoghurt Sauce

(one serving)

2–3 slices	pineapple, peeled and cored
1	banana
$^1/_2$	papaya
$^1/_4$	melon, seeded
1 tsp	honey
1 tsp	lime juice
1 tbsp	butter
1 recipe	Honey Yoghurt Sauce (see below)
to garnish	mint

Honey Yoghurt Sauce Mix together 2 tsps yoghurt, 1 tsp honey, seeds scraped from 1 vanilla bean, 1 gm ($^1/_4$ tsp) ground cinnamon.

Method Cut the fruit into large cubes of equal size and skewer them. Brush them with lime juice and a bit of honey (optional). Then brush with butter and grill. Try to get sear marks from the hot grill. Drizzle the sauce over the skewers and garnish with sprigs of mint.

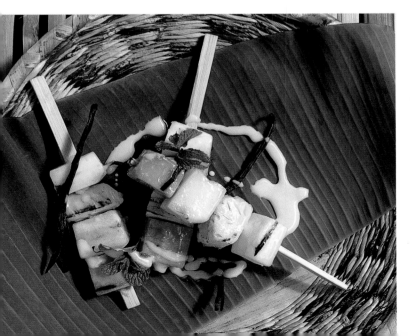

Liquid Assets

Everybody knows that healthy eating is a metaphor for feeling great and living longer but the adage "you are what you drink" hasn't caught on with the same fervour. The daily prescription for two litres of water somehow never makes the leap from our minds to our gullets. But it is in fact drinking good quality fluids regularly that has the most important impact on our general health. And it doesn't just have to be water – spring, filtered or distilled. Here are some other options:

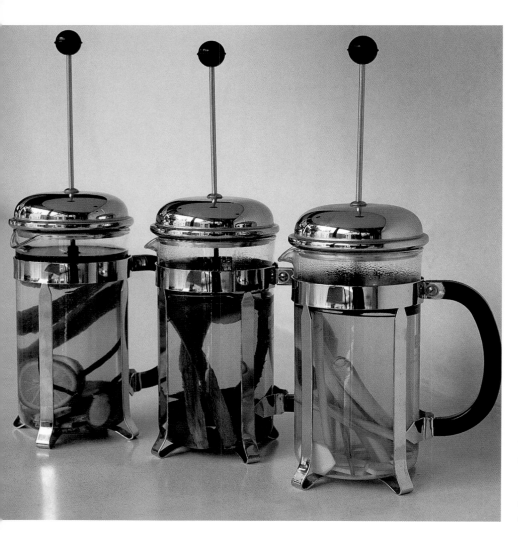

Herbal teas and freshly squeezed juices inject us with just as much vitality as health-giving foods. Such fluids flush out unwanted toxins and help re-hydrate the body's organs, increasing blood flow and moving oxygen more efficiently around the body. In this respect they are ideal for topping off the benefits of a body treatment or massage.

Natural juices and smoothies, containing yoghurt or milk with puréed fresh fruit, have become part of the healthy eating lexicon because they are excellent meal substitutes and that much more easy to digest than solid foods. They are perfect spa food because they satisfy our mild hunger pangs after treatments without overloading the system. Fruit, in particular, is easily digestible and cleansing while containing fructose, which gives energy. It also has a cooling, calming action on the body and has that all-important high water content.

Both fruit and vegetables are important sources of anti-oxidant vitamins and minerals which zap free radicals, those harmful molecules that damage cells and cause premature ageing and such conditions as cancer, heart disease, arthritis and diabetes. The most important vitamins found naturally in fruits are vitamins A, C and E. But besides all its health giving properties, fruit, whizzed into a thick, tangy pulp, with or without milk and yoghurt, is so deliciously refreshing that it's usually gone in a gulp.

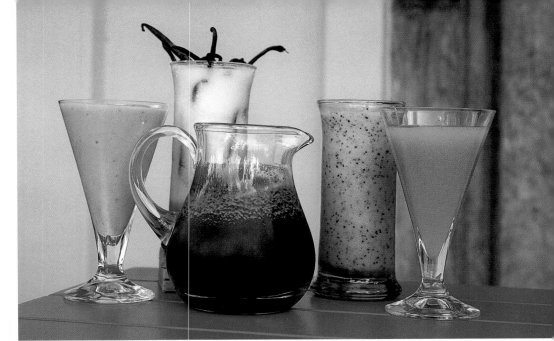

Herbal Infusions

Herbal teas started with the Greeks and Romans and were drunk all over the world until the 1940s when Western medicine became overrun with science and frowned upon any alternative approach. By contrast, infusions of herbs and spices have always had a role in oriental diet for the mild effect they can have on stimulating the kidneys, calming digestion, aiding circulation and, of course, putting water back into our bodies (this we apparently lose at a rate of 1.8 litres per day).

Discard the dusty tea bags that start off bland and become stale in favour of loose-leaf herbs and spices in their natural state. You can concoct a variety of teas to suit your mood and your taste buds. Try some camomile for stress, nettle for skin problems, garlic or peppermint for bronchitis, ginger for tummy trouble and raspberry leaf in preparation for labour.

Some popular infusions from *The Serai* in east Bali are pictured left:

Ginger and lemon grass – a stomach settler and tonic for pregnant women; it also helps with motion sickness.
Cinnamon, ginger and lime leaf – for warming the body in cool weather, with mild astringent properties.
Vanilla, cinnamon, lime fruit, turmeric and ginger – ginger and turmeric are blood cleansers and stomach settlers; the vanilla adds flavour and the lime has acidic and cleansing properties.

Thirst-Quenchers

From *The Spa at Jimbaran*, Four Seasons Resort, Bali

Tropical Passion – passion fruit, orange, banana and lime juice
Coconilla – cool coconut water and milk with vanilla beans
Blushing Beat – beetroot, cucumber and fresh lime
Guava Gulp – mango, guava nectar, banana and lime juice
Jamu Wanita – Javanese herbal drink believed to clean the blood, improve vitality and act as an aphrodisiac!

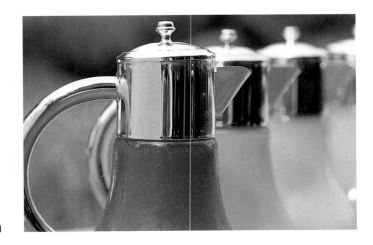

Just Juices

From *The Datai*, Langkawi

Watermelon juice, Orange juice, Guava juice and Melon juice.

Herbal Tonics

Jamu is one of the greatest success stories of the beauty industry, yet it is virtually unknown outside its country of origin, Indonesia. In that country, 80 percent of the population relies on its natural medicinal powers to attain the figure, the complexion, the physical strength or the mood they desire. Broadly speaking, jamu refers to any kind of traditional medicine. But most people think of jamu as a herbal beverage with medicinal qualities and swig back a daily glass to achieve their heart's desire – or a few more glasses to cure an ailment already there.

The origins of jamu are lost in time, though, like most of the country's beauty rituals, it is supposed to have been born in the in central Java where commercial production is still based. The purest forms of jamu come from the island of Madura, where women reputedly can live to 135 years of age.

In fairytale fashion the magic jamu potions – herbs, roots, barks, leaves, honey, fruits, egg yolk and 'other ingredients' – are handed down verbally from mother to daughter through the generations. It is very much a woman's industry.

While the more common mixtures are taken for general health, strength and beauty, there are more than 350 well-known recipes for conditions as varied as skin whitening, kidney stones, malaria and flu. Most popular jamus contain turmeric for its astringent qualities and tamarind for flavour and blood cleansing. The dried ingredients are usually mixed with water plus a little honey or lime to taste. Under commercial production, the potent plant matter is ground into powder and pill form for convenience. However, a bag of dried herbs from Madura still has the greatest effect and stays potent for five years.

Visit *Hotel Tugu* in Bali for access to the best jamu available (see recipes below and right). Not only does this spa have a hot line to Madura, they make the traditional tonics on site. Most of Indonesia's spas offer more palatable jamus for general wellbeing. Drink one before or during your treatment to warm and prepare your body.

Jamu Koeat Lelaki (Strong Man Jamu)

This is a man's jamu. It makes one glass. It is taken to enhance vitality and endurance in bed. For continual high performance, a glass should be drunk morning and evening.

1 tbsp	black pepper, crushed
1 tbsp	coffee beans, ground
100 gms (2 tbsp)	ginger juice, from soaked, shredded ginger
3 tbsp	honey
juice of 1	lime, juiced
1	free-range egg

Method Put all the ingredients into a glass and mix. Cover with half a glass of hot water and drink down immediately.

Jamu Koenci Seoroeh

This is a women's jamu: it eliminates body odour, reduces the intensity of both period and period pains and is taken to keep the body tight and youthful. It can be drunk, like water, any time. The following recipe makes five bottles of jamu, or three days supply.

200 gms (1 cup)	Chinese keys (*Boesenbergia pandurata*)
100 gms (6 tbsp)	galangal (or ginger)
100 gms (6 tbsp)	turmeric, ground
3 tbsp	coriander, ground
handful	betel leaves (*Piper betle*)
200 gms (1 cup)	pressed tamarind
500 gms (1 lb)	coconut sugar
150 gms (6 tbsp)	white sugar
3 litres (3 quarts)	drinking water
to taste	salt

Method Clean, peel and cut the Chinese keys, galangal and turmeric. Put these together in a juicer with the coriander and betel leaves and water. After blending, strain. Soak the tamarind in warm water and strain it to get the juice. Mix the coconut sugar and white sugar together in boiled water and strain. Combine all the above in a bowl and add salt to taste before serving. The amount produced can be kept for up to one week in the fridge.

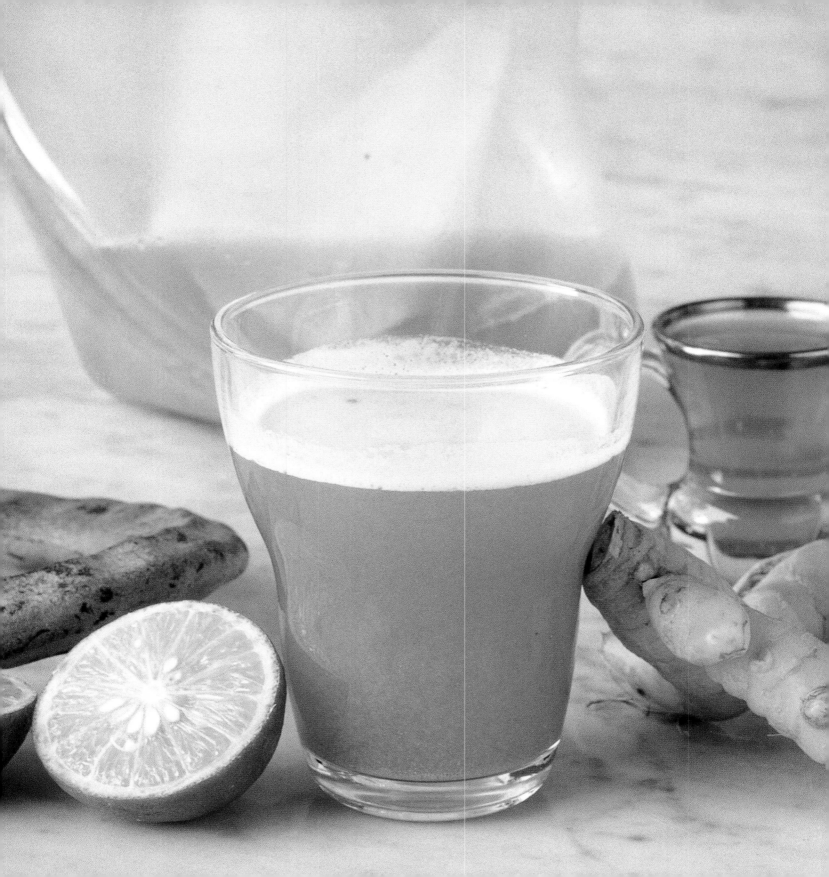

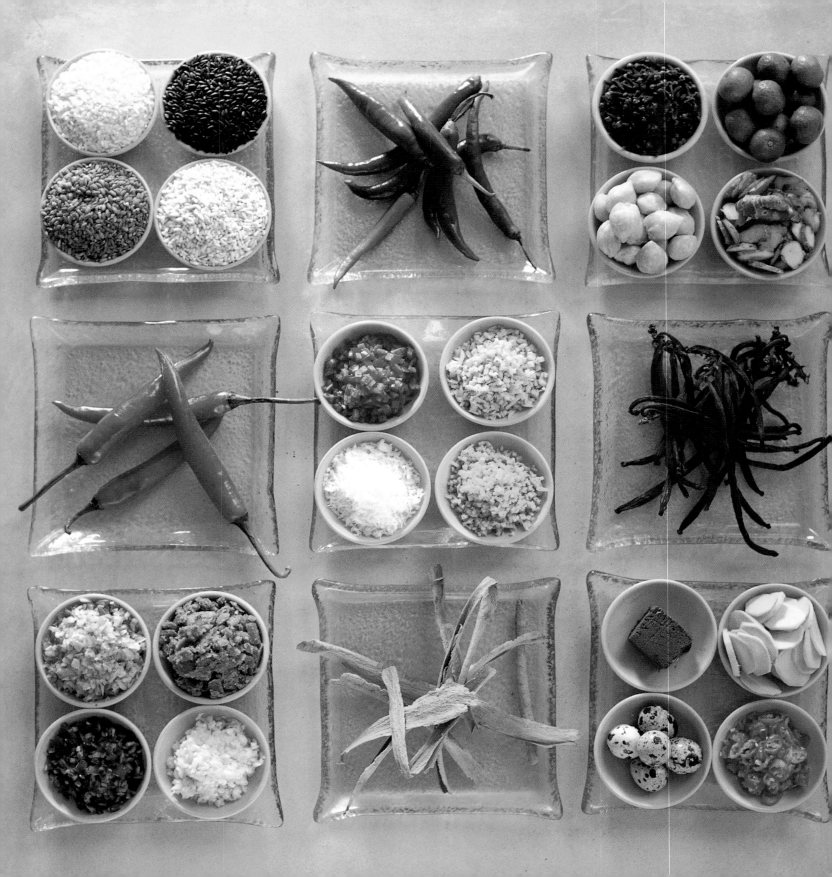

natural spa ingredients

The enormous wealth of natural eco-systems makes southeast Asia a botanical treasure trove. The medicinal qualities of much of its abundant plant life have, for centuries, formed the backbone of health and beauty therapy throughout this huge and exotic continent. Such is the potency of nature in this part of the world that it has found favour in beauty salons everywhere. Here we list some of the most common natural ingredients used.

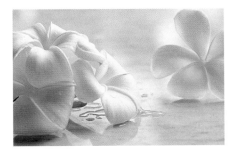

FRANGIPANI or PLUMERIA (*Plumeria sp.*) is one of the most prolific flowers in tropical Asia. The waxy, aromatic blooms fall constantly from the tree of the same name; consequently, they are commonly used in offerings and ceremonies and to decorate religious icons. The plumeria tree is often planted on grave sites in the region.

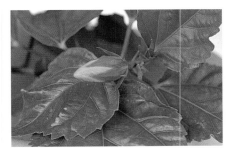

The HIBISCUS LEAF (*Hibiscus sp.*) is the sole ingredient of a traditional form of shampoo. When they are crushed and boiled in a little water, the leaves' sap forms a sticky, dark-coloured paste that has cleansing properties. The leaf has also traditionally been used as a cleanser in a variety of skin care preparations.

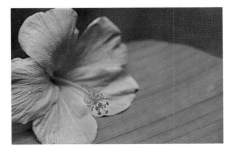

HIBISCUS FLOWERS (*Hibiscus sp.*) are believed to hold certain supernatural powers which absorb negativity and bad spells. The traditional red, orange, yellow and pink blooms have a sweet nectar. They are used for ornamentation purposes and are often found on religious statues. They are also used as an emollient in skin care.

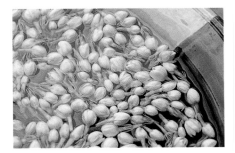

JASMINE (*Jasminum sp.*) is another of tropical Asia's most sweet-smelling flowers. In Thailand, it is a symbol of friendship, and is often strung into garlands and offered to people as a welcome gift and to Buddha as a sign of gratitude. This tiny bud is woven into hair for wedding ceremonies in Java.

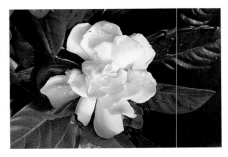

TROPICAL GARDENIA (*Gardenia jasminoides*) is regarded almost as an emblem of the tropics, due to its beautifully strong aroma. In many tropical Asian households, the blooms are put in a bowl of water and displayed in the home where their strong scent permeates into the environment.

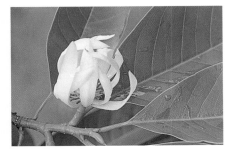

TROPICAL MAGNOLIA or CHAMPAK (*Michelia champaca*) is renowned for its cooling and healing powers with specific anti-malarial properties. Its petite web of elegant white petals exudes a scent as sweet as syrup. Like most of her sisters, it is used in prayer ritual and for bathing.

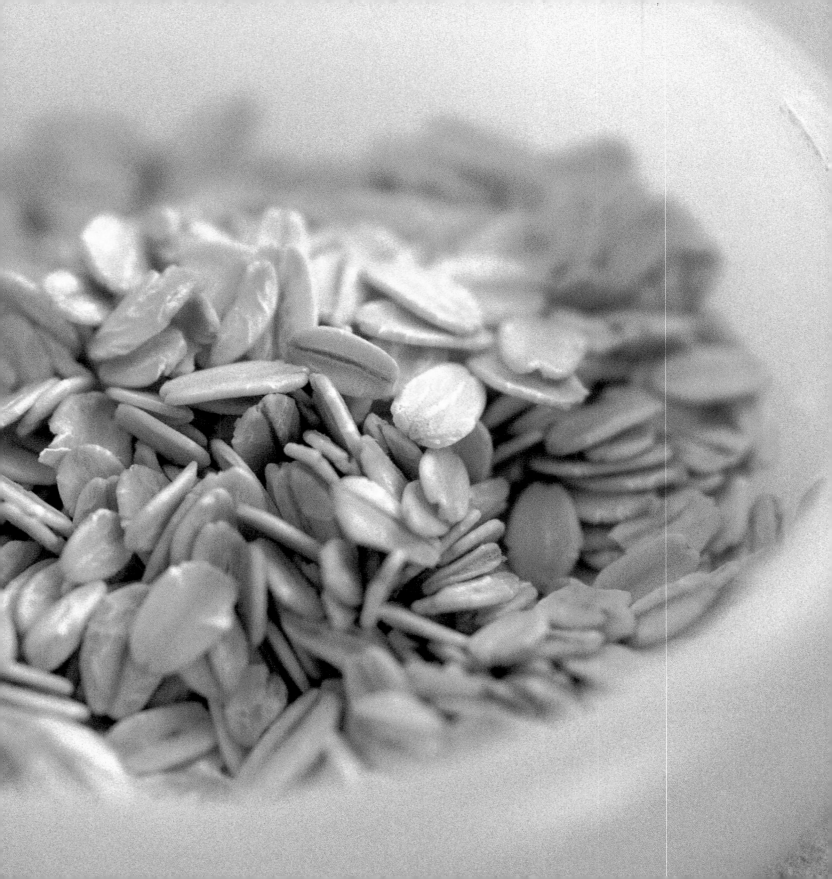

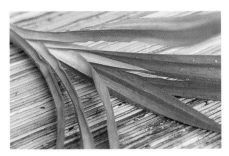

PANDANUS LEAF (*Pandanus amaryllifolius*) is a versatile leaf grown in most gardens, *apotik hidup* (which translates as the 'healing pharmacy') in Indonesia. Thanks to its earthy and sweet aroma this practical leaf is a popular base for cakes and is infused into oils for hair and skin care. It is also used in virtually all Balinese offerings to the Gods.

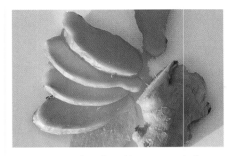

GINGER (*Zingiber officinale*) is eaten cooked or infused raw into drinks, as a remedy for stomach aches and menstrual pains. Myth says that ginger is key to assisting man's endurance in love-making due to the phallic shape of the rhizome! Used externally, ginger is applied to the body to relieve aching muscles and increase blood circulation.

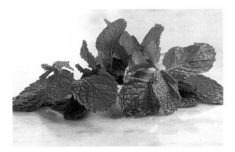

MINT (*Mentha arvensis*) is a blood cleansing plant because it is antiseptic and antibacterial. It is most commonly taken as a tea simply by infusing a few leaves in boiling water, in order to help clear the complexion. It is also mixed with the crème bath conditioner and rubbed into the scalp to combat dandruff and stimulate hair follicles for growth.

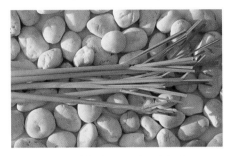

LEMON GRASS (*Cymbopogon citratus*) is a key flavouring in Asian cuisine, resembling lemon rind more closely than the juice. The swollen base of the stem is used, but the whole stalk should be soaked before use. It is eaten to speed up a slow digestive system; its oil is good for calming hot, perspiring feet. Burn the oil for an effective room deodorizer.

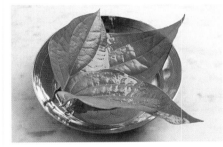

BETEL LEAF (*Piper betle*) is an astringent leaf, associated with feminine cleanliness: it is used as a sanitary wipe and as a cleanser when added to bath water. The fresh leaves are cooling on a hot body. It makes a bitter tea believed to help 'dry the vagina' and purify the blood. Both the nut and the leaf are also chewed for a mild stimulating effect.

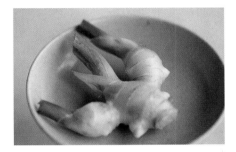

GALANGAL (*Alpinia galanga*) is a rhizome in the ginger family. It has a complex and earthy taste and a pungency and tang quite unlike common ginger. It is most commonly used in cooking, but its faint aroma of camphor makes it one of the spices used in traditional, warming body scrubs such as the Indonesian *boreh*.

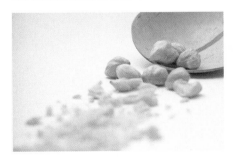

CANDLENUT (*Aleurites moluccana*) is used in cooking across the Asian region. In skincare, the nut's soft and oily consistency makes it a wonderful 'scrub' ingredient. It also acts as soap because, when rubbed over the skin, it draws out impurities and, as proof, changes from creamy to dirty in colour.

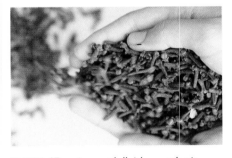

CLOVES (*Eugenia caryophyllus*) have analgesic qualities and are traditionally used for pain relief, especially for toothache. They are also antiseptic, increase overall blood circulation and, when chewed, can stop excessive flatulence! Suck a clove when you are tired or stressed or want to give up smoking.

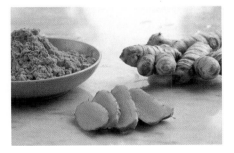

TURMERIC (*Curcuma domestica*) is a basic item in folk medicine in tropical Asia. It is used internally and externally for its astringent and cleansing properties and is a core ingredient for jamu herbal tonics in Indonesia. Its vivid colour gives the Javanese *lulur* (body scrub) its signature orange hue.

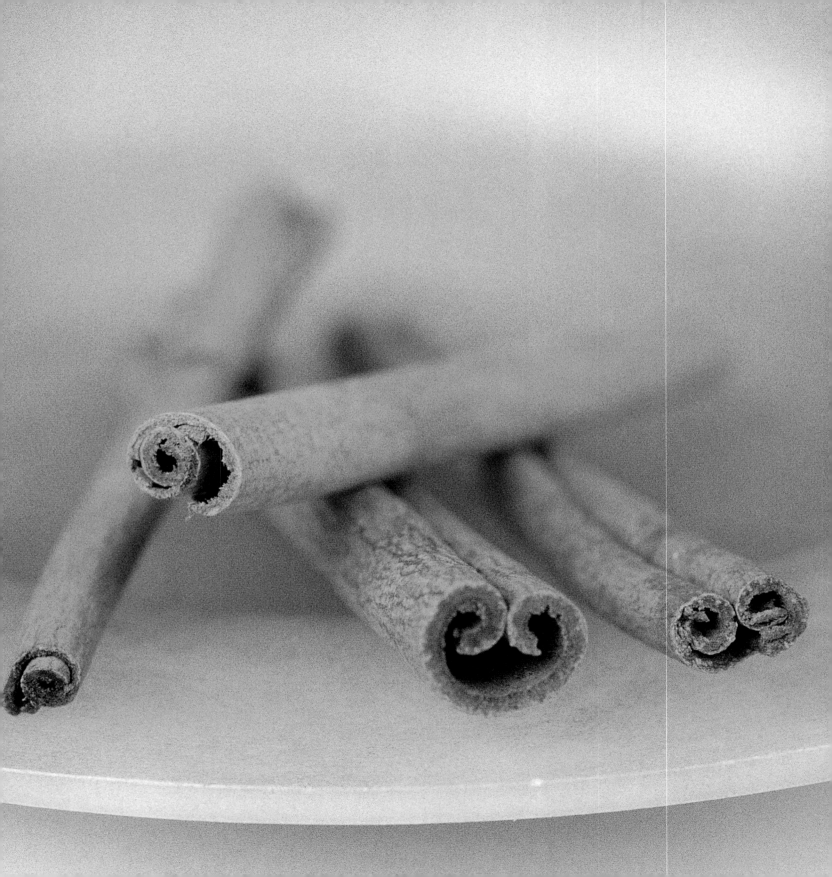

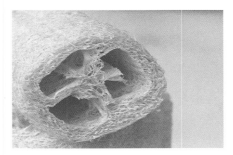

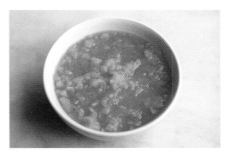

CUCUMBER (*Cucumis sativus*) is used extensively in beauty products as a cooling and revitalizing agent, and is especially effective for oily skin types: its juice makes a good skin tonic and tightens the pores. Cucumber slices on the eyes refresh and moisturize and, for those who forgot their SPF, mashed cucumber soothes sunburnt skin.

NATURAL SPONGE, otherwise known as 'loofah', is the dried body of the green *gambas* plant. Its fibrous yet gentle constituency makes it ideal for removing dead skin cells while still softening and refreshing the skin. The loofah body scrub, often combined with sea salt and oil, is popular at Thai spas for those who want to invigorate their skin.

PAPAYA (*Carica papaya*), abundant throughout tropical Asia, contains vitamins (particularly high in A and C) that heal upset stomachs. It contains enzymes which give it mild exfoliating properties, so Asian women daub papaya around their eyes to eradicate fine lines. Alternatively, papaya skins can be rubbed over the face to remove dead skin cells.

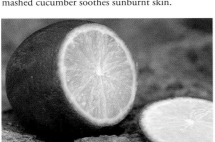

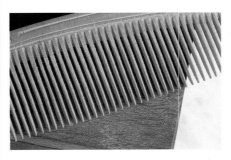

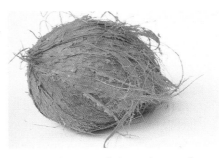

LIME (*Citrus sp*) is used in drinks, food, medicines and beauty regimes throughout southeast Asia. It is high in vitamin C and its astringent qualities make it an effective blood purifier. It is mixed with crushed sea shells and smeared over the stomach as part of traditional slimming ritual and is said to be effective in shrinking the uterus after childbirth.

SANDALWOOD (*Santalum sp*) is the most sacred and fragrant of woods, preserved for burning in temple ceremonies. Its heavy, sweet and woody aroma is instantly recognized. In beauty, it is the hallmark of oriental perfume, although it is also believed to calm skin irritations, such as eczema and abscesses, thanks to its astringent properties.

COCONUT (*Cocos nucifera*) is used in countless ways: for eating, drinking, as an ingredient in cakes and as tropical Asia's most prevalent cooking oil. Oil from mature fruit is massaged into the head for soft and shiny hair while the thick white milk is traditionally used as a shampoo and the young, thin milk as a conditioning rinse.

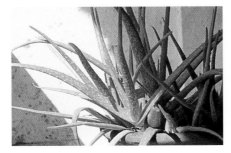

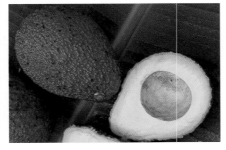

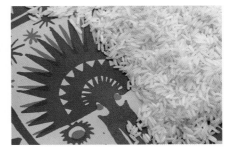

ALOE VERA (*Aloe vera* syn. *Aloe barbadensis*) is much prized for the miraculous healing qualities of the thick, clear liquid stored in its leaves. It is used externally to clear skin blemishes, scars and heal burns or sunburn; internally it may be taken in tablet form for digestive complaints.

AVOCADO (*Persea americana*) is popular in natural beauty practice because the rich consistency of its flesh and oil, high in vitamin E, is a nourishing skin food, especially effective for dry complexions and brittle hair. Avocados were introduced to southeast Asia two centuries ago from America.

RICE is not just a food, it is a culture and a way of life. Paddies dominate the Indonesian landscape where 8,000 varieties are believed to be grown. Rice is food for half the world's population and, in beauty ritual, is used as a base in body scrubs due to its exfoliating properties.

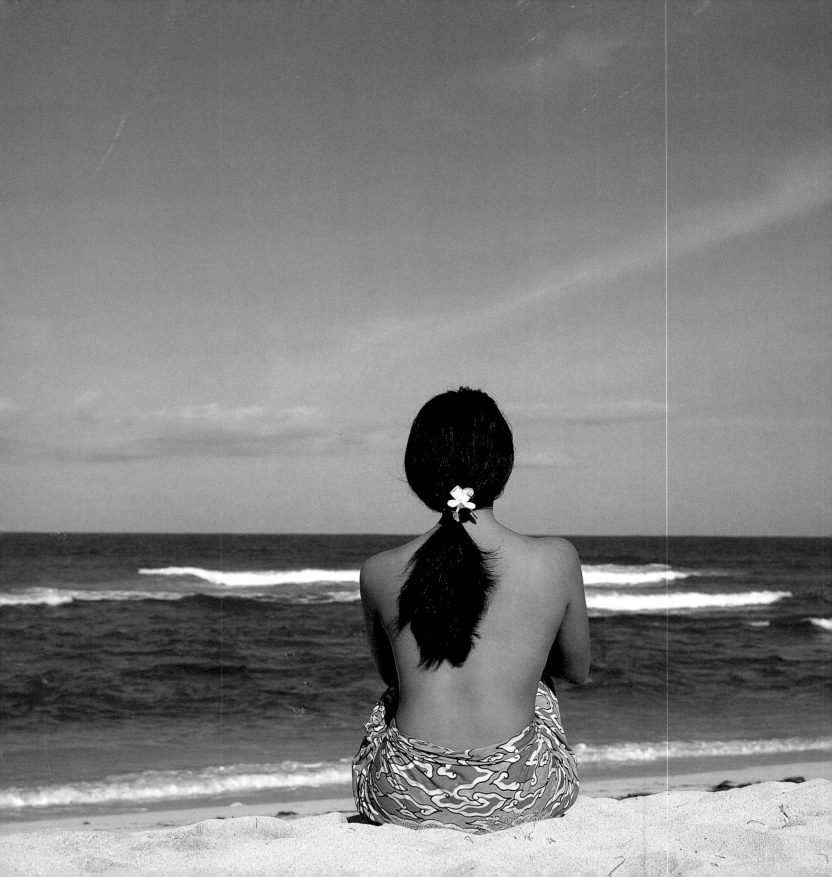